Essential Radiology in Head Injury

Dedication
For Angela, Ian and Katherine
D.W.H. Mok, 1988

Essential Radiology in Head Injury

A diagnostic atlas of skull trauma

D W H Mok

Orthopaedic Registrar, Department of Orthopaedics, St Bartholomew's Hospital, London

and

L Kreel

Visiting Professor, Department of Diagnostic Radiology and Organ Imaging, Prince of Wales Hospital, Hong Kong

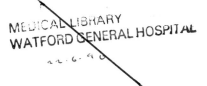

Heinemann Professional Publishing

Heinemann Medical Books
An imprint of Heinemann Professional Publishing Ltd
Halley Court, Jordan Hill, Oxford OX2 8EJ

OXFORD   LONDON   MELBOURNE   AUCKLAND

First published 1988

British Library Cataloguing in Publication Data
Mok, D W H
    Essential radiology in head injury.
    1. Man. Head. Injuries. Diagnosis.
    Radiography
    I. Title II. Kreel, L
    617′.51044

ISBN 0 433 00041 4

Printed in Great Britain by
BAS Printers Limited, Over Wallop, Hampshire
and bound by
Butler & Tanner Ltd, Frome

Contents

Foreword

The curriculum for the training of medical students has undergone many changes over the past few decades, and has become increasingly detailed, complex and overloaded. There are many areas in which teaching is sparse and indeed some of these have considerable importance to the young recently qualified doctor. One such subject is diagnostic radiology. It is appreciated that adequate training in radiological interpretation over all subjects is not possible during the undergraduate years. However, even in the postgraduate years, the junior doctor often finds himself ill-equipped to make a radiological diagnosis. This is seen particularly in accident and emergency departments, where casualty officers are called upon to interpret radiographs, often when no radiological opinion is available. In an analysis of 360 cases of litigation involving radiological interpretation, 78% of cases were related to trauma. By far the most difficult region for radiological analysis is the skull, where the inexperienced have problems even in distinguishing vascular markings from vault fractures.

This book is intended to fill this educational gap and to provide a practical atlas for dealing with head injuries. The authors are experienced in both radiology and in orthopaedics, and trauma surgery. Dr Kreel is a senior and distinguished radiologist of international reputation who has collected impressive material providing many excellent illustrations. Mr Mok has utilised his experience in trauma surgery obtained in many centres, including District General Hospitals, St George's Hospital, London and The Royal National Orthopaedic Hospital, Stanmore. Although this book is intended as an atlas, there are excellent chapters covering the normal anatomy, radiography (including radiographic projections), and describing and illustrating pathological lesions. It is because this is such an excellent book to meet the needs of every casualty officer, and indeed any doctor wishing to practise trauma surgery, that I feel so honoured in giving this foreword.

> J. O. M. C. Craig
> Consultant Radiologist
> Director, Department of Diagnostic Radiology,
> St Mary's Hospital, London
> Past Vice-president, Royal College of Radiologists

Preface

House officers in accident and emergency departments have an extremely onerous task. All over the world the system is similar: junior doctors, usually only one year after graduating, are taken into accident and emergency departments without the necessary preliminary training and are expected to deal with every type of patient, from the most trivial cases to people virtually at death's door. This, of course, was also previously the case in general practice where after the compulsory year of internship, a doctor was considered qualified to care for a whole community. Now, for general practitioners in the United Kingdom, there is a training programme that includes hospital and general practice under the aegis of a senior general practitioner. Clearly, where there is no similar programme for casualty officers they need all the help they can get.

Usually there is little difficulty in calling on surgical and medical registrars and even paediatric and gynaecological registrars, but how frequently after hours can a pathologist's or radiologist's opinion be obtained? It is also unfortunate that in most institutions neither medical nor surgical house staff have been given training in pathology or radiology.

There has, however, been a significant improvement in recent years, with the appointment of consultants in accident and emergency and the emergence of accident and emergency medicine as a specialty in its own right. Undoubtedly these departments and the corresponding hospitals have benefited greatly. What is more, hospital planners have recognized the importance of having accident and emergency cheek-by-jowel with departments of radiology, allowing the development of close cooperation. Consultations between the personnel of the two departments are now frequent, resulting in greatly improved practice and renewed interest in common problems, benefiting patients and doctors alike.

Nevertheless, crucial difficulties persist. The hazards of radiation and the cost of investigations must be among the foremost. Public concern with radiation has in the past been directed more towards nuclear plants and nuclear weapons with a view to preventing contamination of the land, sea and air, but now pregnant mothers frequently question the risk and necessity of any investigation, even sonography. Many patients ask about the risk of radiation from computed tomography and barium examinations. It is time the medical profession as a whole became aware of these concerns.

The cost of investigations must also not be neglected. We are in a period of economic stringency in which the public sector is being severely limited, not least the National Health Service, and radiological examinations are expensive. Yet it is all too easy to fill out or even get a nurse or sister to fill out a request form. Does every injury really need a radiograph? Are there no clinical criteria to distinguish patients who will benefit from those who will not? Or are we to be plagued by the spectre of being sued even when all our training and experience tells us that the radiograph will not make the slightest difference to the way we treat the patient? Does it really alter management actually to see a linear fracture of the base of the fifth metatarsal or of a phalanx of a toe?

There are now recommendations on head injuries backed by both the Royal College of Radiologists and the Royal College of Surgeons and perhaps a start could be made by following these recommendations.

However, radiographs of the skull are difficult to interpret and will continue to be so because of the complex anatomy and the numerous normal variants that can be mistaken for pathology. To add to the difficulty artefacts are commonly present, particularly on skull radiographs for accident and emergency departments, the commonest being blood in the hair. But then there is the discipline of remembering to look at all aspects including the soft tissues, paranasal sinuses and the upper part of the cervical spine visible on the skull film. And how much more difficult for junior house staff in the middle of the night when senior colleagues are not available for consultations. We hope that this book will provide assistance particularly for those sorts of occasions.

If we can add just one more plea. In a head injury, especially in a severe head injury, remember the body that goes with the head. Don't send a patient to a neurological unit without examining the thorax, abdomen and legs. To mix metaphors, it is extremely difficult to get off a 'production line' or a moving bus whose doors are shut. Perhaps one day there will be enough 'trauma units' up and down the country to make such comments superfluous. Until then each district hospital will have overworked accident and emergency departments where the next patient could be one with nothing but skin abrasions or one with a ruptured liver who also has a head injury.

Although modern management of head injuries requires immediate access to computed tomography most district general hospitals, even those with busy casualty departments receiving major trauma cases, do not have the equipment. Obtaining a skull radiograph in some instances will only amount to wasting precious time. A patient at the local hospital who obviously requires a neurosurgical unit can do without a skull radiograph which in any event will almost certainly be repeated at the specialist centre.

Finally, the authors would like to thank the following medical photographers who have put in a lot of effort to provide us with such high quality prints:
Ms Anita Power and Mr Robert Wade of Queen Mary Hospital for Children, Carshalton.
Miss Philpott and Mr Simon Couter of St. James' Hospital, London.
Mr Cook of St. George's Hospital, London.
Mrs N. Hollick of Newham General Hospital, London.

L.K.
D.W.H.M.
London

Chapter 1

Introduction

Head injuries account for at least one million annual attendances at accident and emergency departments in the United Kingdom (Jennett et al., 1977). In the majority of cases, the injury is mild, clinically insignificant and uncomplicated. Nevertheless, skull radiographs are ordered routinely and with alacrity in most casualty departments to determine whether there is a skull fracture, a practice that developed and continues partly because many surgeons and most patients attach great importance to their detection. Junior medical staff have often been taught to associate the presence of a skull fracture with a 200-fold increase in the development of an intracranial haematoma, a condition rightly regarded as an immediate neurosurgical emergency (Galbraith et al., 1981). Furthermore, there is the old medicolegal teaching that every head injury must have a skull examination.

In 1981 the Royal College of Radiologists (RCR) supported a prospective study to investigate the use of skull radiography in the management of patients with head injuries (RCR, 1981). Patients were divided into two categories: complicated head injury, defined as a head injury with additional injury or pathological findings, and uncomplicated head injury, i.e. the rest. The overall occurrence of intracranial haematoma was found to be one in 1207 patients radiographed. In all only four patients had an intracranial haematoma and three of these would have been suspected clinically even if skull radiography had not been available. Therefore at best skull radiography could only have been responsible for alerting the clinician to the possibility of an intracranial haematoma in one of the four cases and the risk of an unsuspected intracranial haematoma with a skull fracture among patients with uncomplicated head injury was one in 4800.

With this data in mind, the RCR in 1983 put forward guidelines for patient selection for skull radiography in uncomplicated head injury which would yield 94% of the vault fractures and all those in whom the outcome was serious (depressed, basal, or frontal fracture, intracranial haematoma, aerocele, or death) (RCR, 1983).

RCR SELECTION CRITERIA FOR SKULL RADIOGRAPHY IN MILD HEAD INJURIES

(1) CSF and/or fluid discharge from nose
(2) Haemotympanum and/or fluid discharge from ear
(3) History of unconsciousness
(4) Altered state of consciousness at the time of examination
(5) Other focal symptoms or signs
(6) Bruising or swelling of scalp

Our recommendations for skull radiography include all children under three years of age who have had skull trauma because one cannot rely on children in this age group to remember the event well enough to estimate the possible extent of the injury and the head injury may be non-accidental.

Over the age of three years, if the head injury was mild, without headache or vomiting and no signs were found on clinical examinations, no radiographic examination is required. A head injury advice sheet should be given to the patient and an additional note should be sent to the general practitioner with information of the event. The patient should return immediately if any untoward signs or symptoms develop.

Moderate head injuries with symptoms and signs conforming with the RCR criteria should have films taken. If the radiographs show the following, the patient should be referred to a specialist unit for a computed tomography (CT) scan.

(1) Fracture across the middle meningeal vascular channel (Fig. 1.1)
(2) Fluid levels indicating a fracture involving the paranasal sinuses (Fig. 1.2)
(3) Gas in the orbit or cranium (Fig. 1.3)
(4) Basal skull fractures (Figs. 1.4, 1.5)
(5) Intracranial or suspected intracranial foreign body (see Fig. 9.31)

Severe head injuries with the following symptoms and signs should be referred to specialist centres with the prospect of a CT scan (Figs. 1.6, 1.7) and no time should be wasted in obtaining plain radiographs of the skull.

(1) Unconscious patients, including unarousable alcoholics
(2) A documented decreasing level of consciousness
(3) Palpable skull depression (Fig. 1.8)
(4) Unexplained neurological signs
(5) Persistent otorrhoea, rhinorrhoea, as well as blood behind the eye with periorbital haematoma, and blood behind one or both ear drums

Casualty officers in The National Health Service in Great Britain are usually quite junior, having taken up the appointment immediately after their pre-registration year and without any formal training in the interpretation of radiographs. As a consequence, undetected fractures or misinterpretation is not too uncommon. Studies have shown a marked deficiency in this regard (de Lacey et al., 1980). Casualty officers cannot easily recognize fractures or distinguish fractures from normal vascular grooves in the cranium. Quite clearly casualty officers must by and large develop a better understanding of the plain radiographs of the skull in acute trauma, be aware of the normal anatomy, artefacts and important abnormalities but also have an overview of the indications and contraindications for requesting skull radiographs.

This book is intended to serve as a practical atlas for dealing with head injuries in accident and emergency departments. The principal aim is to develop a systematic approach to the interpretation of skull radiographs; the book is also a guide to obtaining necessary further views to reach a final diagnosis. The differences between normal variants and pathological findings are shown in each chapter so that the reader is made aware of them.

REFERENCES

de Lacey G., Guilding A., Wignall B., et al. (1980). Mild head injuries: a source of excessive radiography? *Clin. Radiol.*, **31**, 457.

Galbraith S., MacMillan R., Jennett B. (1981). X-rays for skull fractures. *Lancet*, **i**, 272.

Jennett B., Murray A., MacMillan R., et al. (1977). Head injuries in Scottish hospitals: Scottish Head Injury Management Study. *Lancet*, **ii**, 696.

Royal College of Radiologists (1981). Cost and benefits of skull radiography for head injury. *Lancet*, **ii**, 791.

Royal College of Radiologists (1983). Patient selection for skull radiography in uncomplicated head injury. *Lancet*, **i**, 115.

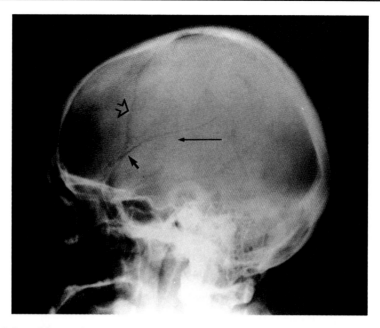

Fig. 1.1a Linear fracture (bold arrow) in frontoparietal region crossing the frontal branch of the middle meningeal vessel (long arrow) as well as a venous channel (open arrow). This should alert the clinician to the possibility of an underlying subdural haematoma and an urgent referral for CT scan is indicated.

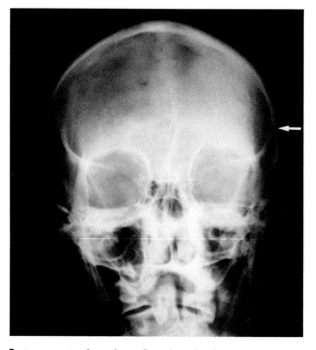

Fig. 1.1b Anteroposterior view showing the fracture line, just visible on the left (arrow).

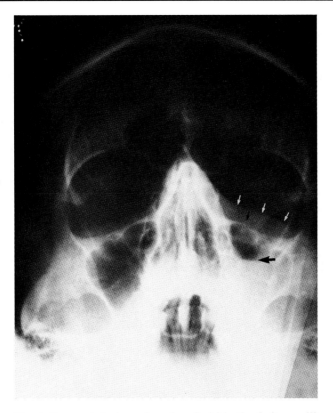

Fig. 1.2a Occipitomental view showing fluid in the left maxillary antrum (bold arrow). There is a blow-out fracture of the left orbital floor (small black arrow) associated with an overlying soft-tissue swelling (white arrows). Direct coronal CT is ideal for the demonstration of the degree of the soft-tissue herniation through the fracture of the anterior orbital floor.

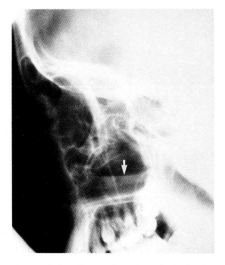

Fig. 1.2b Lateral view of the face showing a fluid level in the maxillary antrum.

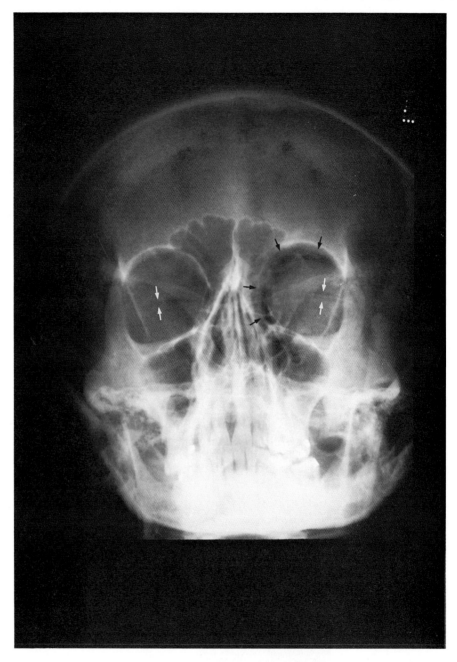

Fig. 1.3   Left orbital emphysema forming a sickle-shaped transradiancy along the superior and medial margin (black arrows). There is also air trapped between swollen eyelids (white arrows).

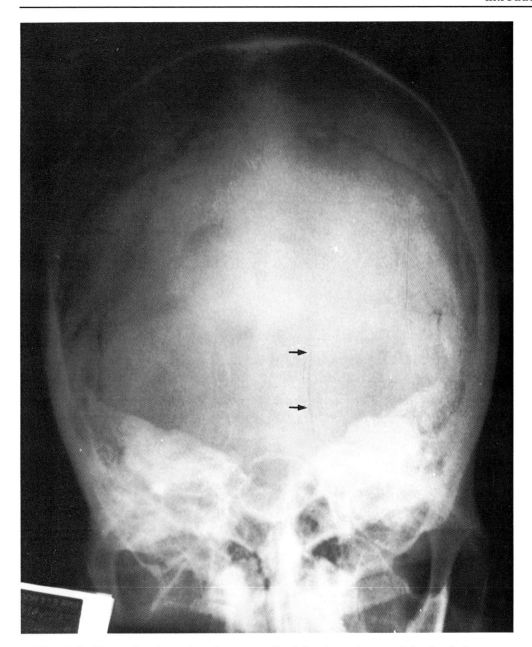

Fig. 1.4 Towne's view showing a vertical fracture (arrows) in the left occipital bone extending onto the foramen magnum. The patient should be referred for a CT scan.

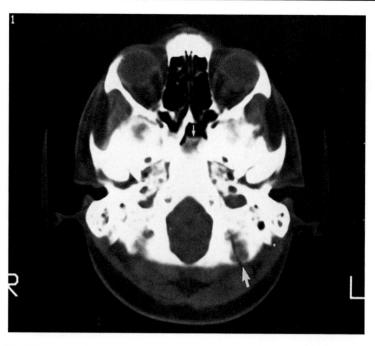

Fig. 1.5 Computed tomography scan of a basal skull fracture (bold arrow) of the left occipital bone also showing a fluid level (small arrow) in the sphenoid sinus indicating involvement of both the posterior and middle fossae. Basal skull fractures are better shown and more readily accomplished on CT than on the basal view with conventional radiography. The basal view must not be done in the acute phase of a head injury.

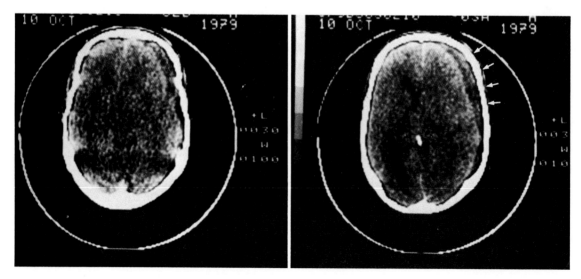

Fig. 1.6 Computed tomography scans showing subdural haematoma on the left (arrows) with marked deviation of the lateral ventricles due to the mass effect of trauma to the adjacent cerebrum.

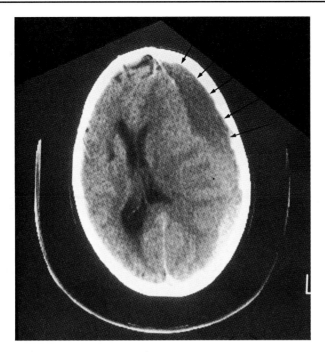

Fig. 1.7a Acute left subdural haemorrhage (arrows) in a patient who was knocked down by a bus.

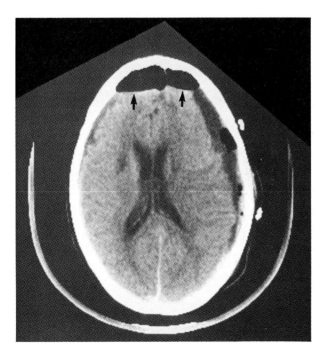

Fig. 1.7b Postoperative CT scan showing that the shift of midline structures has been restored. There is now gas in the cranium with residual blood giving rise to air-fluid levels (arrows).

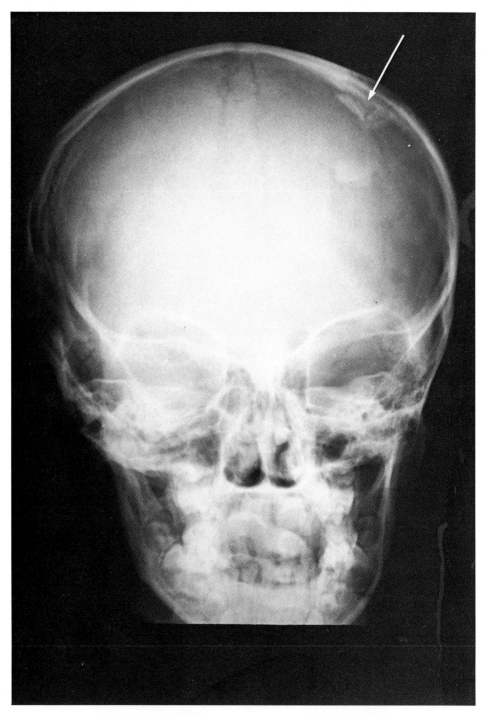

Fig. 1.8a A palpable depression indicates a depressed skull fracture (arrow). This child has a depressed skull fracture in the left parietal region. One fragment of bone has been driven into cerebral tissue necessitating immediate neurosurgical referral.

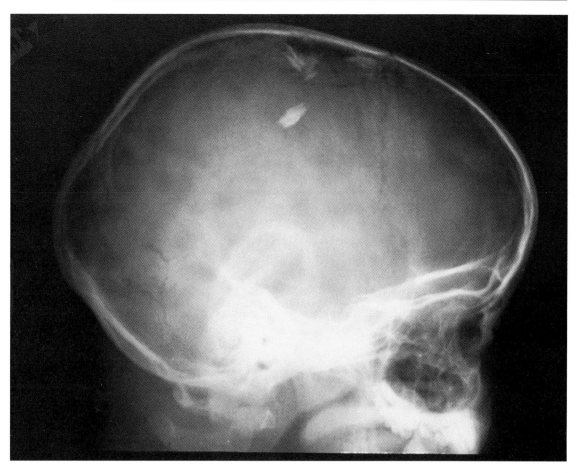

Fig. 1.8b Lateral view of depressed skull fracture showing the extent as well as the depth of the injury in this child.

Chapter 2

Projections and radiological anatomy

The accurate interpretation of skull radiographs requires a detailed knowledge of the normal anatomy, of common variants and of artefacts, particularly in accident and emergency departments where many such examinations are requested daily.

Careful unhurried viewing is obviously essential but if in doubt ask advice from your local friendly radiologist rather than exposing patients to more radiation with views not easy to interpret. There is of course no routine night-time radiological opinion available in this country in most hospitals. Casualty officers are expected to build up their own expertise. A few hints for the over-stretched accident and emergency doctors may be helpful when in doubt.

(1) Consult the radiographer, who frequently has had considerable experience
(2) View the radiograph systematically and do not be in a hurry
(3) View the dark areas with a bright light
(4) After examining the bone, look carefully for soft-tissue swelling, air-fluid levels in the sinuses, gas in the orbits and possible intracranial air
(5) Above all, the clinical state of the patient is paramount

The following initial projections should be taken in acute trauma.

(1) Lateral view required in all cases
(2) Posterior injury – Towne's view or/and
(3) Anterior injury – occipitofrontal view

LATERAL VIEW (BROW UP FOR FLUID LEVELS)

Radiography

The patient lies supine, occiput resting on a non-opaque cushion, with a horizontal beam across the table. The side of the head subjected to trauma should be next to the film. The centring point lies 2.5 cm anterior to the external auditory meatus and 1 cm above the orbitomeatal line (du Boulay, 1980).

Interpretation of the film

This is the most important view. In the National Hospital for Nervous Diseases, the lateral skull radiograph has been recommended as the only film for routine neurological investigations (Moseley, 1987). While not relevant to head injuries, where the problems are decidedly different (as shown earlier) it does however stress the importance of this view.

Following skull trauma, the lateral view may show air-fluid levels in sinuses, or more rarely intracranial air indicating a fracture with potentially serious complications. An adequate film should be centred on the pituitary fossa with the anterior clinoid process and the orbital roofs of each side superimposed and, to stress yet again, must be done with the patient supine and a horizontal x-ray beam.

To view the lateral skull film systematically so as not to overlook air-fluid levels, follow the bony outline of the cranium, scanning both the inner and outer tables of the skull from the occiput to the frontal bone and note the following anatomical landmarks (Figs. 2.1, 2.2, 2.3):

lambdoid and coronal sutures
the grooves of the anterior and posterior divisions of the middle meningeal
    artery
sphenoid sinus
sella turcica
facial structures
upper cervical vertebrae

TOWNE'S VIEW (HALF-AXIAL)

Radiography

The patient lies supine, occiput resting on the table. The x-ray tube is tilted 30° towards the patient's feet, with the centring point at the midpoint between the two external auditory meatuses in the median sagittal plane.

Interpretation of the film

The Towne's projection is particularly valuable for fractures of the occipital bone and the foramen magnum. A good film should have the foramen magnum just visible above the petrous apices and the dorsum sellae should be projected through the foramen magnum.

Check the following structures (Fig. 2.4):

the bony outline of the vault
dorsum sellae
foramen magnum
occipital sutures
calcified pineal – should be central (see Chapter 3)
zygomatic arches

OCCIPITOFRONTAL VIEW

Radiography

Posteroanterior view with face on the film: the tube is tilted 15° from the orbitomeatal plane craniocaudally projecting the tegmen tympani of the petrous temporal over the inferior margins of the orbits and, therefore, the superior and lateral orbital margins and orbital cavities are not obscured.

In a confused or severely injured patient, a frontooccipital view has to be taken. The film is placed under the occiput and the beam directed to the nasion with 20° tilt upwards, i.e. cranially.

The posteroanterior (PA) film (i.e. with the x-ray tube behind the occiput) should be taken whenever possible because structures closer to the film will have better definition and the radiation dose to the eyes is very much less.

Interpretation of the film

The frontal view produces an overall impression of the facial skeleton and the paranasal air sinuses. A correct projection should show the nasal septum in line with the odontoid peg as both are midline structures. The tegmen tympani should be projected below the inferior orbital margins.

Check the following structures (Figs. 2.5, 2.6):

the bony outline of the vault
orbital margins
zygomatic arches
maxilla
mandible

The maxillary antra are not clearly shown on this view as the petrous bones and occiput overlap the maxilla. Occipitomental views are more helpful for facial injuries, producing a much clearer view of the antra, maxilla and zygomatic arches.

ADDITIONAL VIEWS

The following views may be helpful to define a particular fracture if suspected from the initial radiographs.

Occipitomental view

Radiography

The orbitomeatal line is 60° to the horizontal with the central ray at right angles to the film projected through the nasal cavity. This view is also known as the chin-nose view, i.e. the head is tilted back so that the chin and the nose both touch the film cassette.

Interpretation of the film

The facial skeleton and maxillary antra are clearly demonstrated because the base of the skull is displaced downwards (Fig. 2.7). Firstly, the radiograph should be viewed from a distance and the orbits compared. The antra are normally transradiant (dark) being filled with air.

The five lines of the facial contour should be followed systematically

(McGrigor and Campbell, 1950) (Fig. 2.7b). In most centres, however, this film is taken with the mouth open in order to see the sphenoidal sinus. In this case only four lines are shown. The fifth line, which usually follows the inferior mandibular margin, is then not demonstrated.

Finally, the lucency of the maxillary antra including possible fluid levels should be assessed. If an antrum is opaque, a fracture must be suspected even if a fracture line cannot be identified and must be taken as indirect evidence for such a fracture even though antral fluid could be due to incidental sinusitis.

Tangential view

Radiography

A tangential beam is thrown across the part of the injured skull or area under suspicion.

Interpretation of the film

This view eliminates any overlying shadows that may be confusing but is particularly useful to show displacement in depressed skull fractures (Fig. 2.8).

The basal view

Radiography

The head is placed in hyperextension so that the orbitomeatal plane is as parallel to the film as possible. The x-ray beam is then angled 5° towards the head and centred on the midpoint of a line joining the angles of the mandibles.

Interpretation of the film (Fig. 2.9)

This is known also as the submentovertical view. While this may produce a clear view of the base, it should not be done in acute head injuries particularly those likely to involve the base. Computed tomography not only shows the fractures more clearly but does not require the difficult head manipulations of the submentovertical projections (Figs. 2.10, 2.11).

REFERENCES

du Boulay G. (1980). *Principles of X-ray Diagnosis of the Skull* 2nd edn. London: Butterworths.

McGrigor D. B., Campbell W. (1950). The radiology of war injuries. *Br. J. Radiol.,* **23**, 685.

Moseley I. (1987). Interpreting the skull X-ray. *Br. J. Hosp. M.,* **37(4)**, 340.

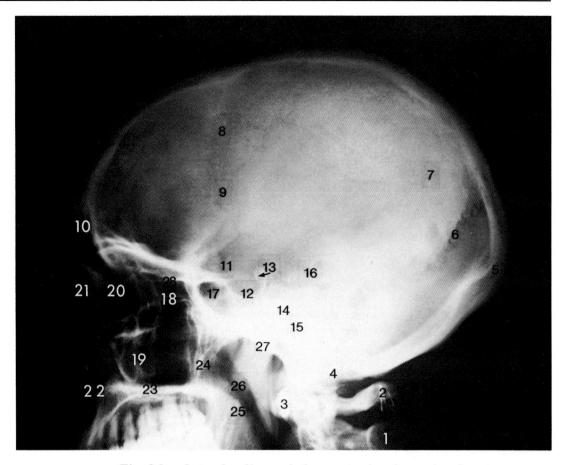

Fig. 2.1a   Lateral radiograph demonstrating the regional anatomy.

1. Posterior spinous process of axis (C2)
2. Posterior arch of atlas (C1)
3. Anterior arch of atlas (C1)
4. Posterior margin of foramen magnum
5. Occipital protuberance*
6. Lambdoid suture*
7. Posterior diploic veins
8. Coronal suture*
9. Anterior diploic veins
10. Frontal sinus
11. Anterior clinoid
12. Floor of the sella turcica
13. Posterior clinoid
14. Clivus (see Fig. 2.2)
15. External auditory meatus (see Fig. 2.2)*
16. Pinna (see Fig. 2.3)
17. Sphenoidal sinus
18. Roof of maxillary antrum
19. Body of the zygoma
20. Orbital cavity
21. Nasal bones
22. Anterior nasal spine
23. Hard palate
24. Pterygoid process
25. Soft palate
26. Nasopharynx
27. Mandibular condyles
28. Ethmoid air cells
29. Squamoparietal suture*
30. Pterion*
31. Greater wing of sphenoid*
32. Temporal bone (squamous part)*
33. Occipital bone*
34. Lambda*
35. Parietal bone*
36. Bregma*
37. Frontal bone*
38. Glabella*
39. Maxilla*
40. Mandible*
41. Mastoid suture*

*On Fig. 2.1b.

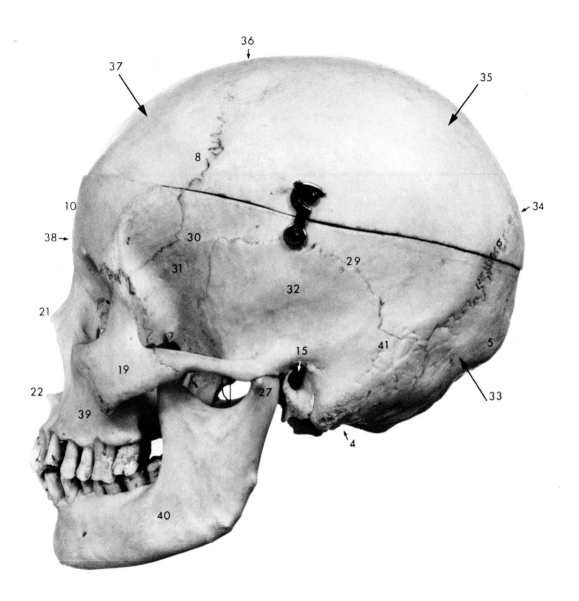

Fig. 2.1b   Regional anatomy of the skull (for key see Fig. 2.1a).

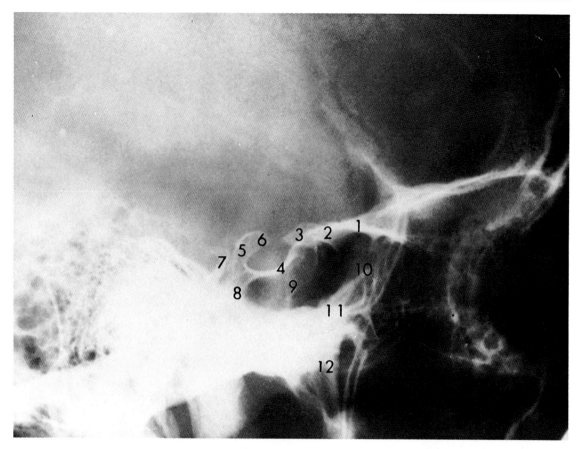

Fig. 2.1c   Lateral view 'coned' onto the pituitary fossa demonstrating the anatomy of the region.

1. Planum sphenoidale
2. Tuberculum sellae
3. Anterior clinoid process
4. Floor of sella turcica
5. Dorsum sellae
6. Posterior clinoid
7. Petroclinoid ligaments
8. Posterior wall of sphenoid sinus
9. Sphenoid sinus
10. Anterior wall of sphenoid sinus
11. Floor of middle fossa
12. Posterior margin of maxillary antrum

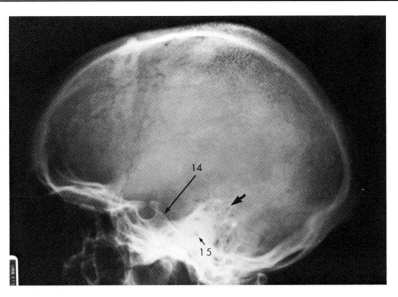

Fig. 2.2   Normal lateral view demonstrating the following anatomical structures:

14. Clivus
15. External auditory meatus   Mastoid air cells (bold arrow).

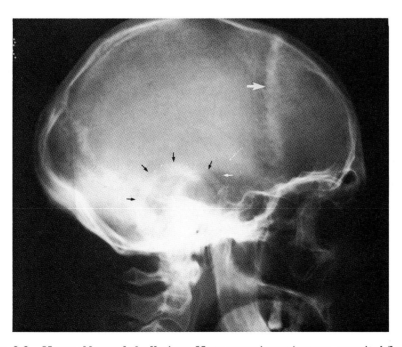

Fig. 2.3   Normal lateral skull view. Note prominent 'suture opacity' (bold arrow) due to bone condensation at the frontoparietal suture and the marked sharp condensation at the frontoparietal suture and the marked sharp groove of the superficial temporal artery (small white arrow). The pinna (black arrows) are particularly well demonstrated here.

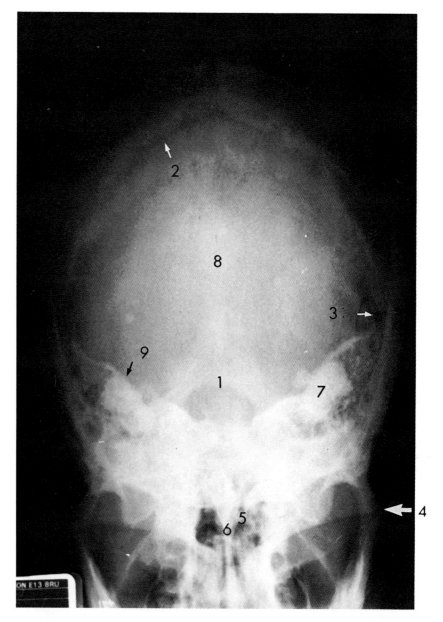

Fig. 2.4a Towne's view: the dorsum sellae can be seen through the foramen magnum.

1. Posterior margin of foramen magnum
2. Lambdoid suture
3. Squamooccipital suture
4. Zygomatic arch
5. Nasal cavity
6. Nasal septum
7. Internal auditory meatus
8. Internal occipital protuberance
9. Tegmen tympani

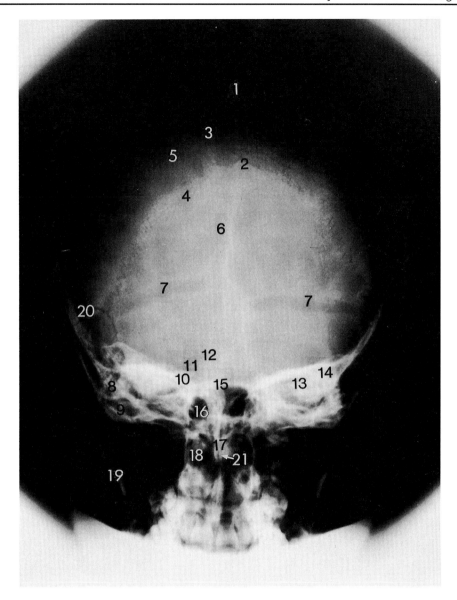

Fig. 2.4b Undertilted Towne's view. The anatomy of the middle ear is shown particularly well on this projection.

1. Sagittal suture
2. Lambdoid suture
3. Bregma
4. Lambdoid suture
5. Coronal suture
6. Sagittal sinus
7. Transverse sinus
8. Mastoid process
9. External auditory meatus
10. Internal auditory meatus
11. Anterior clinoid
12. Posterior clinoid
13. Cochlea
14. Semicircular canal
15. Floor of the sella
16. Superior concha
17. Nasal septa
18. Inferior concha
19. Ramus of the mandible
20. Squamoparietal suture
21. Dens of axis

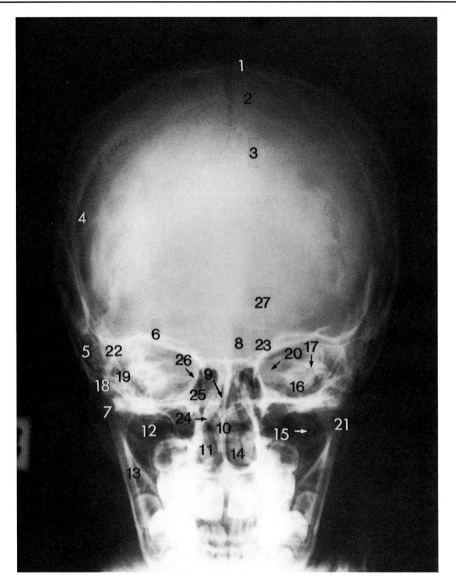

Fig. 2.5a   Occipitofrontal projection (for key see Fig. 2.5b).

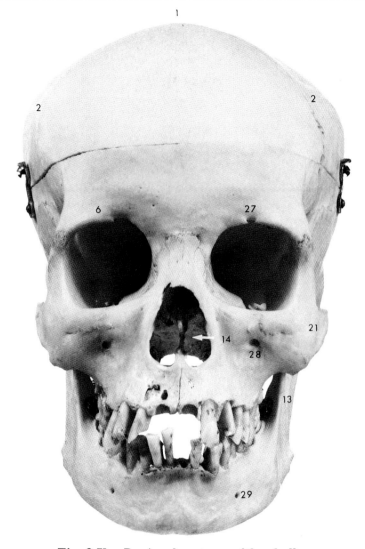

Fig. 2.5b   Regional anatomy of the skull.

1. Sagittal suture
2. Coronal suture
3. Lambdoid suture
4. Lamina interna
5. Mastoid air cells
6. Supraorbital margin
7. Condyle of the mandible
8. Crista galli
9. Sella turcica floor
10. Nasal septa
11. Concha
12. Zygomatic arch
13. Ramus of the mandible
14. Nasal cavity
15. Maxillary sinus
16. Cochlea

17. Semicircular canals (arrow)
18. External auditory meatus
19. Medial margin of external auditory meatus
20. Internal auditory meatus
21. Zygomatic arch
22. Innominate line
23. Anterior clinoid process to lesser wing of sphenoid
24. Ethmoid (posterior air cells)
25. Ethmoid (anterior air cells)
26. Medial orbital margin
27. Supraorbital foramen
28. Infraorbital foramen
29. Mental foramen

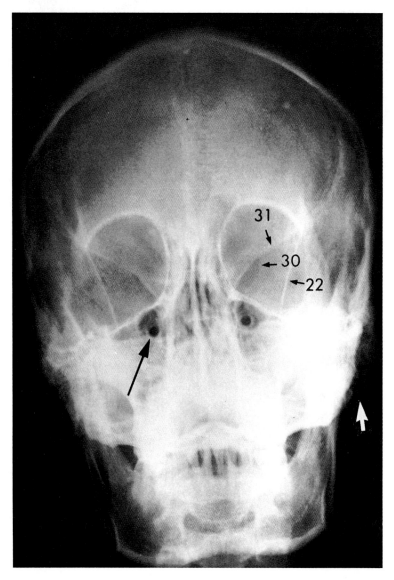

Fig. 2.6 Normal anteroposterior (AP) view of skull demonstrating the following anatomical structures.

22. Innominate line
30. Superior orbital fissure
31. Lesser wing of sphenoid
Foramen rotundum (long black arrow) is
in the body of the sphenoid and transmits
the maxillary nerve.
Mastoid air cells (white arrow).

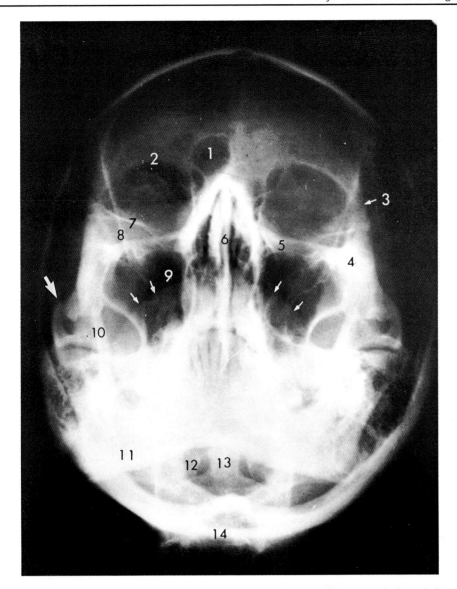

Fig. 2.7a Occipitomental (OM) view showing a fracture of the right zygoma (large arrow). Note the following anatomical landmarks. The soft-tissue shadow of the upper lip (small arrows) curves across the lower margins of the maxillary antra and must not be confused with fluid levels or antral mucosal thickening.

1. Frontal sinus
2. Superior orbital margin
3. Frontozygomatic suture
4. Body of the zygoma
5. Inferior orbital margin
6. Nasal septum
7. Lesser wing of sphenoid
8. Innominate line
9. Maxillary antrum
10. Coronoid process of the mandible
11. Mandible
12. Atlas
13. Dens of axis
14. Margin of the posterior cranial fossa

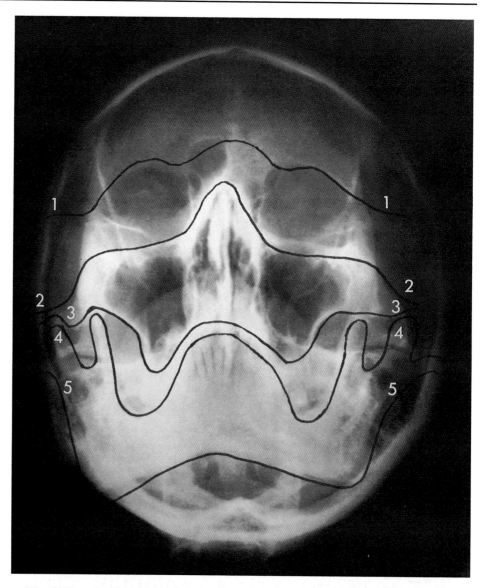

Fig. 2.7b   On the OM view, the five lines for observation of facial symmetry are drawn. If these lines are followed, the fracture in the right zygoma is easy to detect.

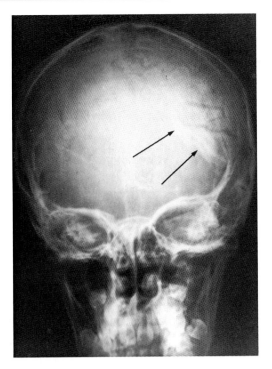

Fig. 2.8a   The frontal view shows the features of 'white line' depressed fractures but the degree of depression is not clearly demonstrated.

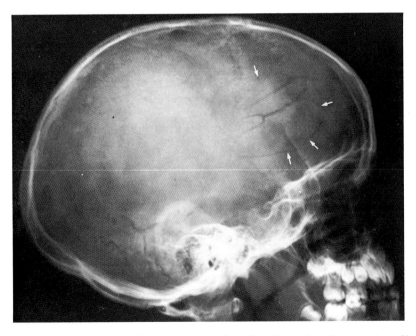

Fig. 2.8b   Comminuted fracture associated with a circular surrounding fracture in the frontoparietal region indicating there is bone depression (arrows).

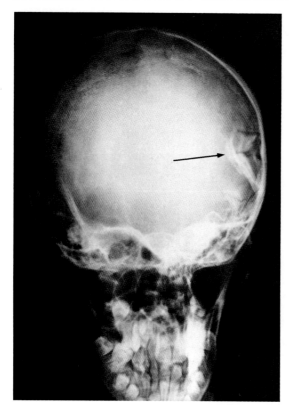

Fig. 2.8c   The degree of depression of the involved bone is now more obvious. Note again the 'white line' fracture (arrow).

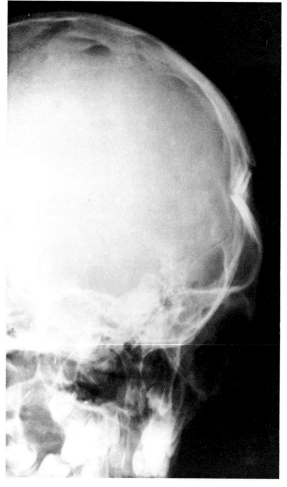

Fig. 2.8d   The true tangential view clearly shows how deeply the bone fragments have been driven below the normal cranial contour.

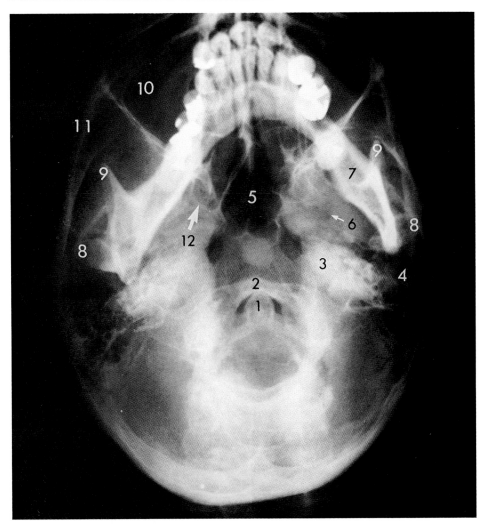

Fig. 2.9   Basal (submentovertical) projection.

1. Odontoid peg
2. Arch of atlas
3. Petrous temporal
4. Mastoid air cells
5. Sphenoid sinus
6. Foramen ovale
7. Mandible
8. Condyle of the mandible
9. Coronoid process of the mandible
10. Overlying orbit and maxillary antrum
11. Zygomatic arch
12. Pterygoid plate

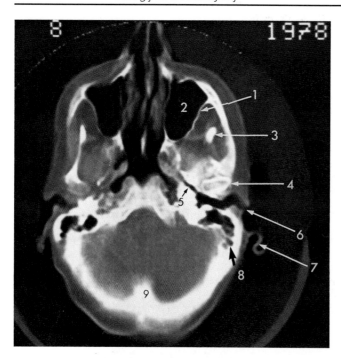

1. Lateral wall of maxillary sinus
2. Maxillary sinus
3. Coronoid process of the mandible
4. Condyle of the mandible
5. Eustachian tube
6. External auditory meatus
7. Pinna
8. Mastoid air cells
9. Internal occipital protuberance

Fig. 2.10   Computed tomography scan demonstrating basal skull view.

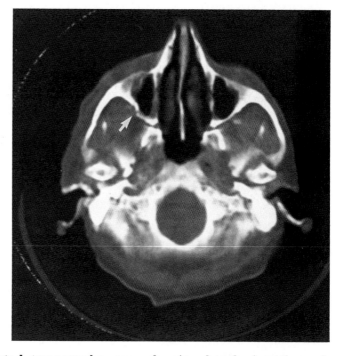

Fig. 2.11   Computed tomography scan showing basal view through maxillary antra with a fracture in the lateral wall (arrow) on the left.

Chapter 3

The calcified pineal gland and other intracranial calcifications

Computed tomography scans are more reliable and efficient than plain radiographs in diagnosing intracranial haematoma, making displacement of the pineal of limited value. However, in the initial assessment in casualty, pineal shift still remains a useful sign as a pointer to intracranial pathology. Shift of the pineal can be due to displacement by a space-occupying lesion, such as a subdural haematoma and associated oedema or due to cerebral atrophy of the opposite hemisphere.

The pineal gland is calcified in 50–70% of adults and this can also occur in children, but if under ten years old rare pineal tumour should be suspected. The calcified pineal may consist of a single nodule or a collection of specks smaller than 1 cm in diameter. Calcified structures in this region larger than 1 cm in diameter are usually pathological (e.g. pinealoma, or aneurysm of the great vein of Galen).

NORMAL POSITION OF THE PINEAL GLAND

In the lateral skull projection (Figs. 3.1, 3.2), the pineal usually lies about 5 cm vertically above the external auditory meatus. The pineal may be displaced upwards and downwards along with tentorial herniation of the brain but the assessment of pineal displacement on the lateral projection is usually difficult without the use of charts (Vastine and Kinney, 1927). More importantly, if the calcified gland is not seen on the lateral view, it will not be seen on any other view as the skull tables are thinner over the temporal region compared with the frontal and squamous occipital bones in the AP projection.

Other normal calcified structures in this area include the glomus of the choroid plexus of the lateral ventricles posteriorly and the habenular commissure anteriorly.

The choroid plexus can readily be distinguished from the pineal on the frontal and lateral projections because on the frontal view they lie well away from the midline (Figs. 3.3–3.7) while on the lateral view the habenula usually forms an incomplete calcified circle immediately anterior to the pineal calcification. To the untrained eye, the difference between the calcified habenula and the pineal may not be obvious; this is an inconsequential distinction as displacement usually affects both equally.

In the axial views, the pineal lies within 3 mm from the midline (Fig. 3.8). Measurement should be taken from the inner table of the skull to the centre of the gland on either side. Displacements from this position are nearly always due to a space-occupying lesion or unilateral brain atrophy.

CALCIFICATION OF THE CHOROID PLEXUS

This can be seen in 75% of adult skull radiographs, on almost all CT scans (Fig. 3.9) but is uncommon in children. The calcifications are usually symmetrical, bilateral and of equal density but recognition of this displacement is difficult on plain radiographs as the position of the posterior part of the normal lateral ventricle can be extremely variable.

OTHER NORMAL CALCIFICATIONS

These include calcification in the falx (Figs. 3.10–3.13), often asymmetrical, attached to one side of the midline and having a peak which protrudes between the cerebral hemispheres. Calcification of these normal structures should be readily distinguished from other intracerebral calcifications associated with cranial pathology (see Fig. 3.21).

Calcification at the base of a parasagittal meningioma may closely resemble falx calcification (Fig. 3.14). Meningiomas of the middle fossa, and particularly those which arise from the petrous apex, may produce an unusually dense collection of calcification in the tentorial attachment and in the petroclinoid ligaments of the same side. Overlying osteoma on the outer table of the skull (Fig. 3.15) may present as a confusing opacity on the lateral view and may require further views to establish the diagnosis.

Long-standing subdural haematomas resulting from head injury as well as from a ruptured aneurysm may calcify, appearing as an incomplete shell conforming to the general shape of the fluid collection.

Calcifications are also quite frequently found in and around the sella turcica, particularly in the petro- and interclinoid ligaments (Fig. 3.21) and in carotid

Similarly calcification can occur in a subaponeurotic haemorrhage forming a calcified shell on the external cranial margin, around the haematoma and later being incorporated into the bone to form localized bone thickening (Figs. 3.17–3.20).

Calcifications are also quite frequently found in and around the sella turcica, particularly in the petro and interclinoid ligaments (Fig. 3.21) and in carotid arteries of elderly persons. Craniopharyngioma, predominantly a childhood tumour, also forms calcifications in the region of the sella.

However, by far the commonest area of increased skull density is the quite benign hyperostosis frontalis interna. On the lateral view, there is a homogeneous density within the frontal bone with a characteristic wavy pattern of curved lines on the frontal view (Figs. 3.23–3.27). The centre of the frontal bone remains unaffected producing a transradient pathway through the denser bone.

REFERENCE

Vastine J. A., Kinney K. K. (1927). The pineal shadow as an aid in the localisation of brain tumours. *Am. J. Roentgenol.*, **17**, 320.

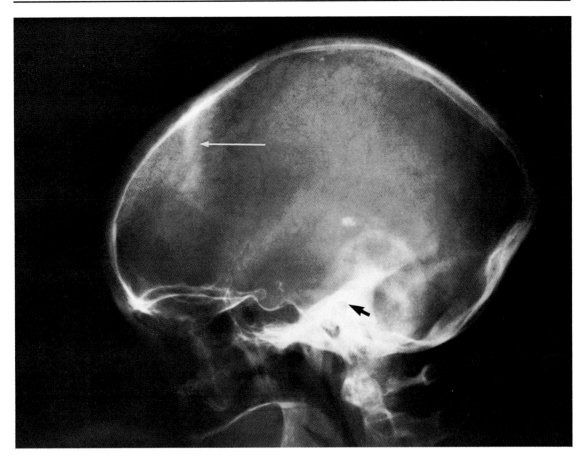

Fig. 3.1 Normal pineal calcification lying directly above the external auditory meatus (black arrow). The bone density adjacent to the bregmatic suture (white arrow) is a common normal variant.

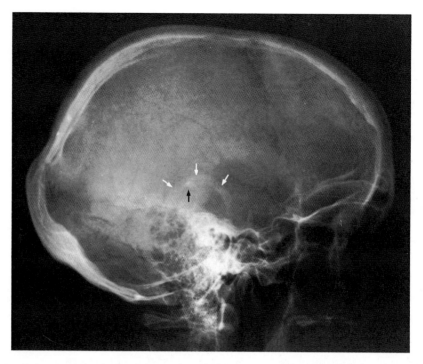

Fig. 3.2 Calcified pineal on a lateral film demonstrating its normal position. The curvilinear shadow of the pinna (white arrows) overlies the pineal calcification (black arrow).

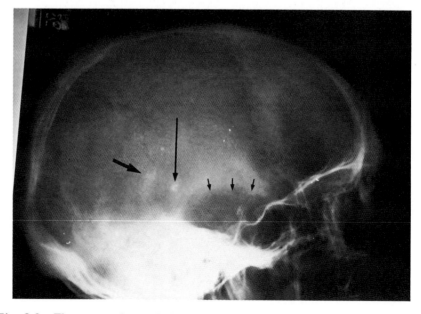

Fig. 3.3 The posterior relationship of the calcified choroid plexuses (bold arrow) to the pineal (long arrow). The dark lower part of the squamous temporal bone (small arrows) is a normal variant.

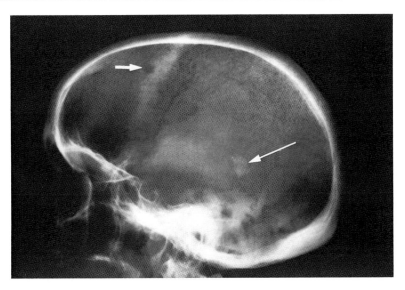

Fig. 3.4a Marked choroid plexus calcification demonstrated (long arrow). There is also a small venous lake just anterior to the bregmatic suture (short arrow). Note that the pineal is not calcified in this case.

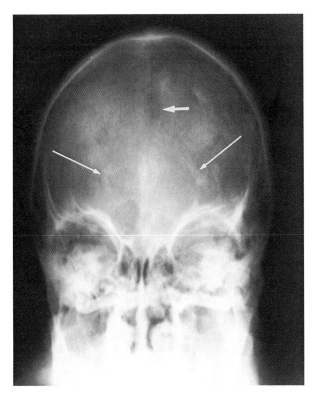

Fig. 3.4b Occipitofrontal view showing marked calcification in the choroid plexus (long arrows). The venous lake (short arrow) is a common normal variant particularly in the occipital bone.

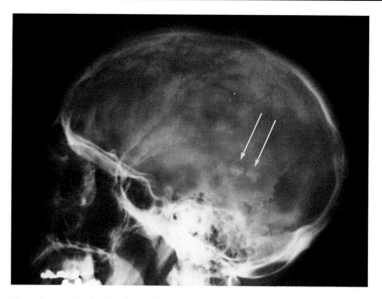

Fig. 3.5a   Lateral skull view demonstrating both calcified choroid plexuses (arrows). This radiograph also shows another normal variant, namely the 'digital type' impression in the cranium producing areas of transradiancy adjacent to denser areas of bone.

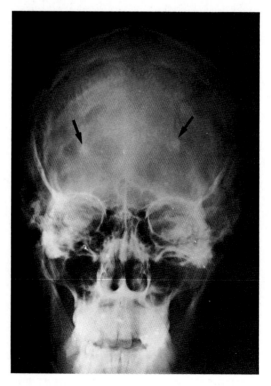

Fig. 3.5b   Occipitofrontal view of the calcified choroid plexuses. The asymmetry is a not uncommon normal variant.

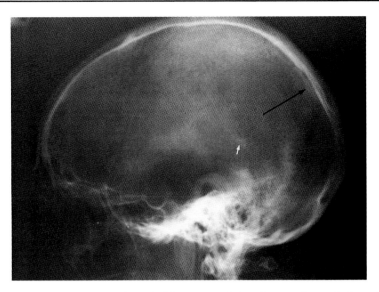

Fig. 3.6a Faint calcification (white arrow) in the region of the pineal gland due to choroid plexuses, also seen on the occipitofrontal view. There is also faint calcification in the posterior aspect of the falx (black arrow).

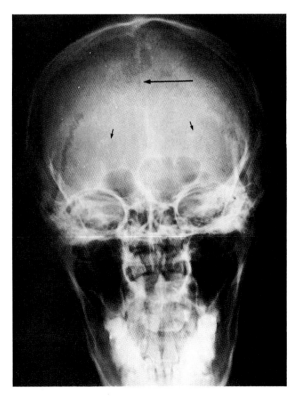

Fig. 3.6b Faint calcifications just visible well away from midline positions due to choroid plexuses (small arrows). The falx calcification (long arrow) is in the midline.

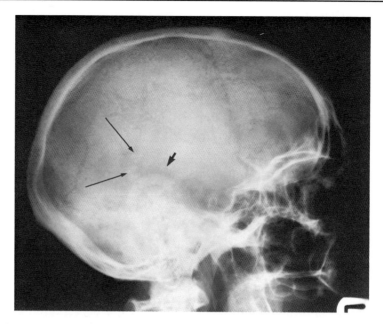

Fig. 3.7   Lateral view showing normal venous channels, normal sclerosis of the frontoparietal suture and calcification of the choroid plexuses (long arrows) and pineal (short arrow).

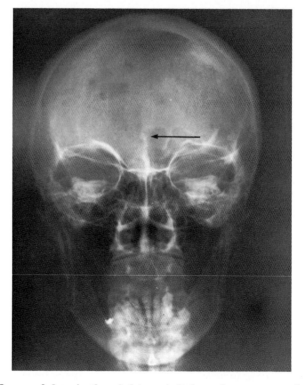

Fig. 3.8   Venous lakes in the right occipital region must not be mistaken for osteolytic defects. Note the central position of the pineal (arrow).

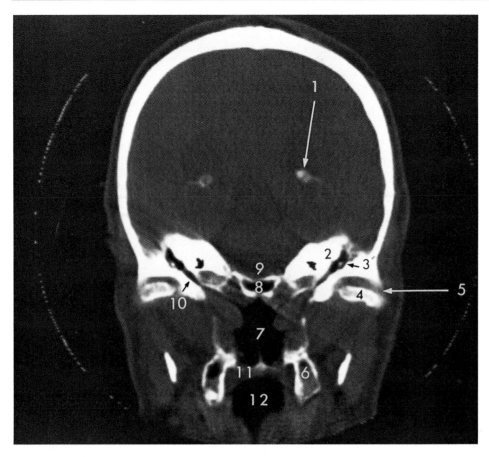

Fig. 3.9 Computed tomography scan of coronal section demonstrating the following anatomical landmarks.

   1. Calcified choroid plexus
   2. Apex of petrous temporal
   3. Middle ear ossicle
   4. Condyle of the mandible
   5. Temporomandibular joint
   6. Pterygoid process
   7. Nasopharynx
   8. Posterior aspect – sphenoid sinus
   9. Floor of pituitary fossa
  10. Eustachian tube
  11. Hard palate
  12. Oropharynx

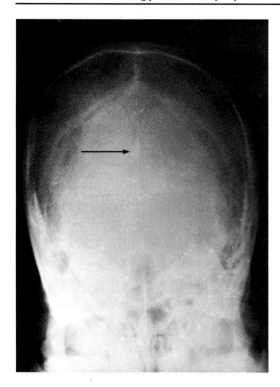

Fig. 3.10a Towne's view showing normal calcification of the falx (arrow). The calcification is asymmetric, with a straight midline edge on the left but protruding laterally on the right – a not uncommon normal variant.

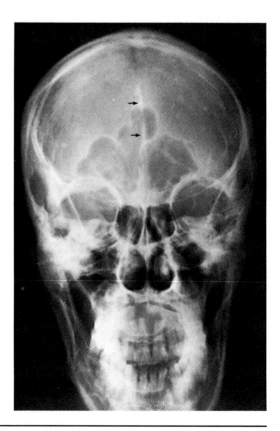

Fig. 3.10b Calcified falx (arrows) in midline projected over the superior part of the frontal sinus.

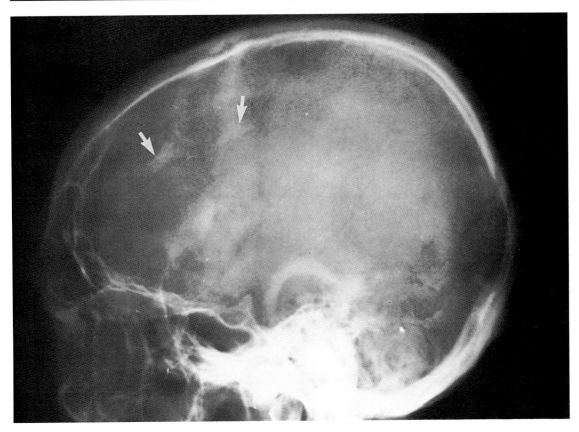

Fig. 3.10c The calcified falx on the lateral view is not as easily recognized, often producing confusing shadows if not related to a frontal projection.

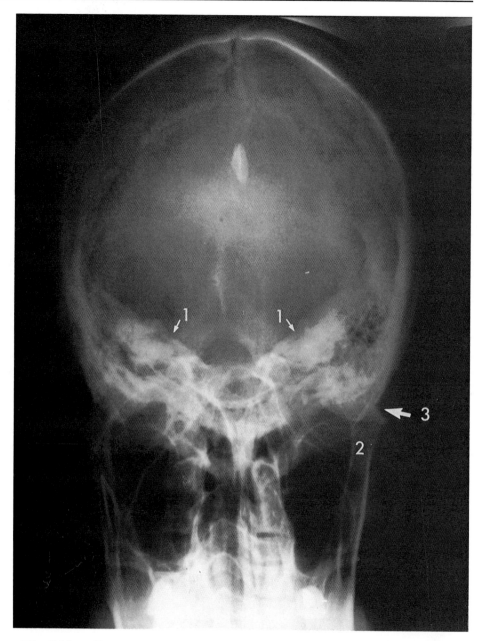

Fig. 3.11a   Towne's view showing a midline calcification of the falx with symmetrical widening. The internal auditory meatuses (1) are well shown on this view as well as the mandibular condyles (2) and temporomandibular joints (3).

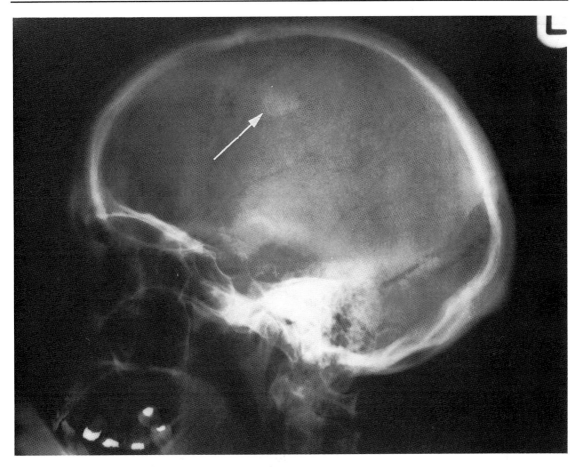

Fig. 3.11b Lateral view of Fig. 3.11a showing the calcification is in the falx (arrow).

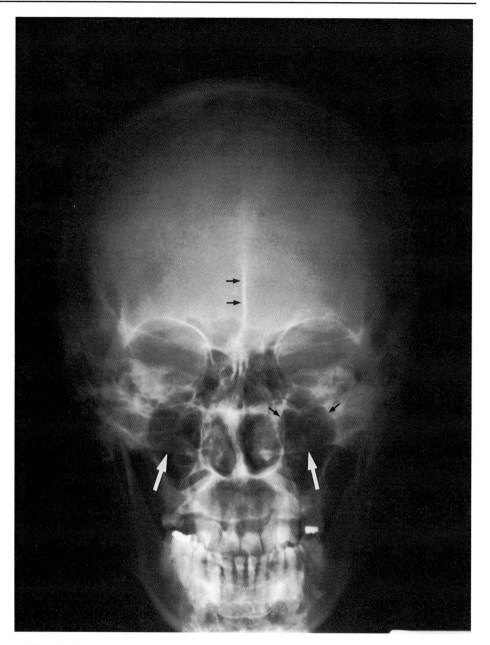

Fig. 3.12 Occipitofrontal view showing calcified falx as a central thin white line (black arrows). The maxillary antra (black arrows) are displayed but projected over the transverse lines of the posterior fossae at the skull base (white arrows).

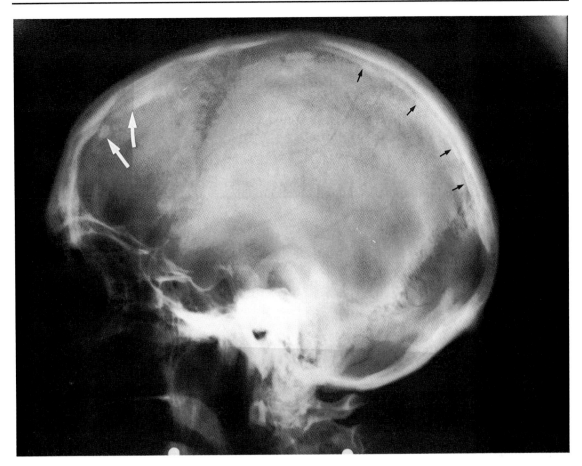

Fig. 3.13 Lateral view of a patient with calcification in the frontal region (white arrows) in the falx and along the margin adjacent to the inner table of the skull (black arrows).

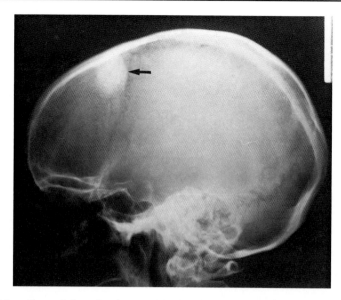

Fig. 3.14a Round density (arrow) in the frontal region with the base adjacent to the inner table in a meningioma.

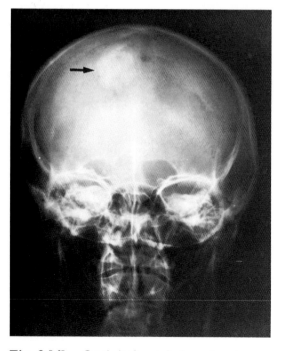

Fig. 3.14b Occipitofrontal view showing the calcification (arrow) associated with a frontal meningioma.

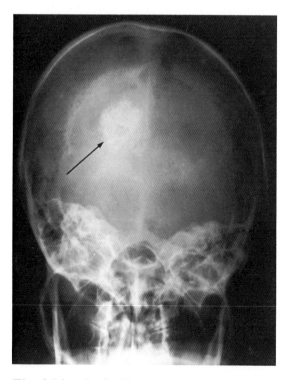

Fig. 3.14c In the Towne's view, the frontal meningioma (arrow) can be seen to be adjacent to the falx.

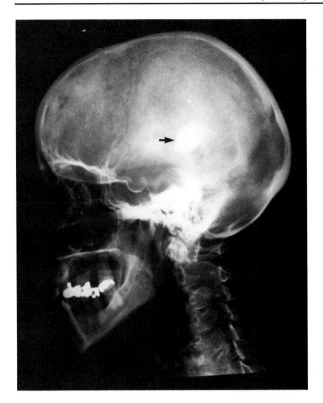

Fig. 3.15a The rounded density (arrow) in the posterior parietal region must be localized on a frontal view for diagnosis. The small lucencies in the frontal region are due to Pacchionian granulations.

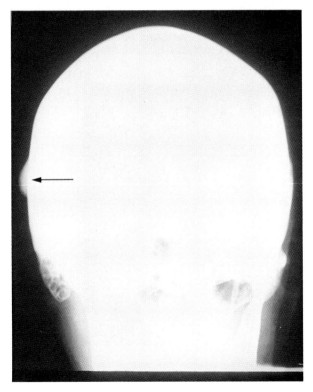

Fig. 3.15b The tangential frontal view demonstrates well the osteoma on the outer table (arrow).

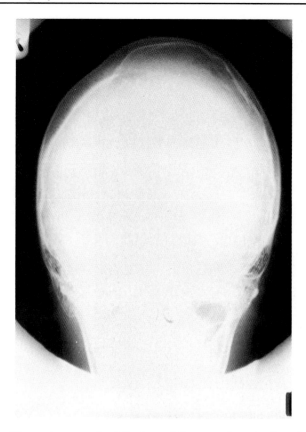

Fig. 3.16a   There is a marked bulge of the cranium in the right parietal region due to bone expansion around an extradural haematoma.

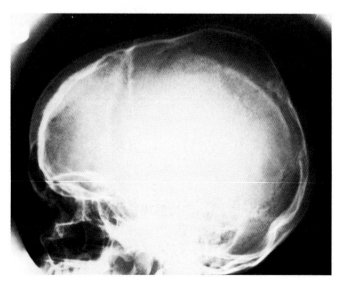

Fig. 3.16b   The lateral view shows a similar appearance, with the outer table expanded over the old extradural haematoma.

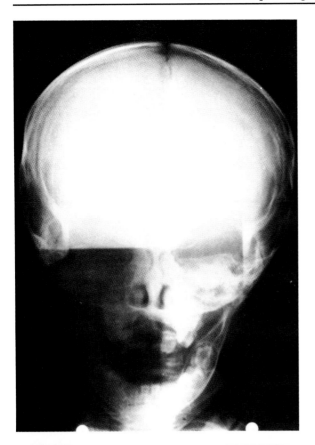

Fig. 3.17 Frontal view of a child, showing an exposure artefact of the right side of the face but no fracture or other abnormality. However, viewing the film with a bright light showed a subaponeurotic haematoma.

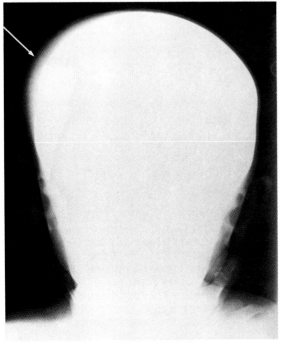

Fig. 3.18 Subaponeurotic haematomas are usually not well demonstrated with routine exposures and require a bright viewing light to identify the lesion. A soft-tissue exposure will however demonstrate the subaponeurotic haematoma (arrow).

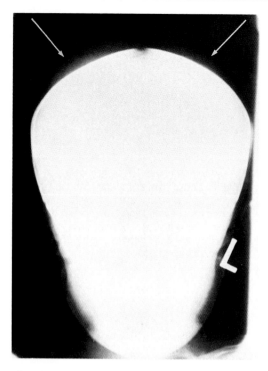

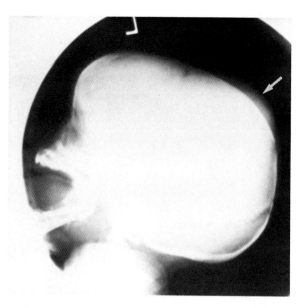

Fig. 3.19a Soft-tissue exposure demonstrating subaponeurotic haematomas (arrows). Note that in infants the haematomas are bilateral.

Fig. 3.19b The parietal subaponeurotic haematomas also shown on the lateral soft-tissue film (arrow).

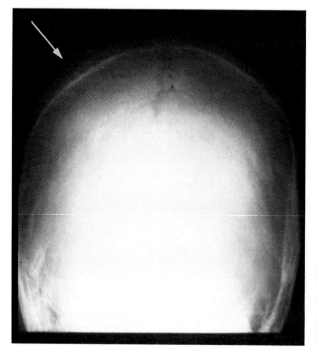

Fig. 3.20 Old subaponeurotic haematoma (arrow) which has calcified and has subsequently been incorporated into the bone to form localized bone thickening. The appearance of old subaponeurotic and extradural haematomas can easily be distinguished by the position of the margins of the skull tables; below is subaponeurotic and above is extradural.

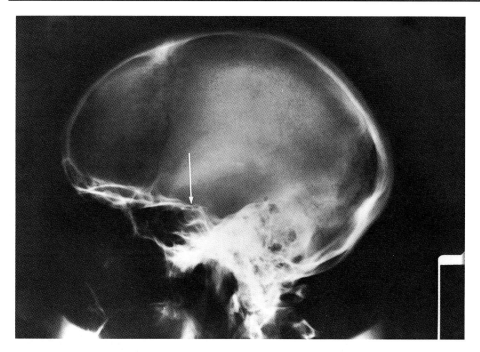

Fig. 3.21a Lateral view showing interclinoid calcifications forming a 'roof' for the sella (arrow).

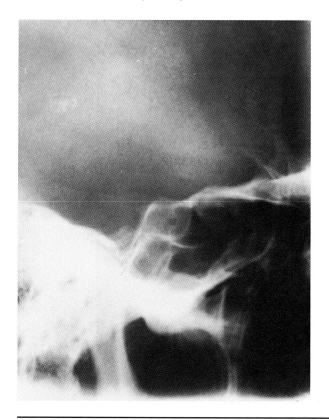

Fig. 3.21b Coned view of pituitary fossa showing calcification in the interclinoid ligaments forming a roof across the sella.

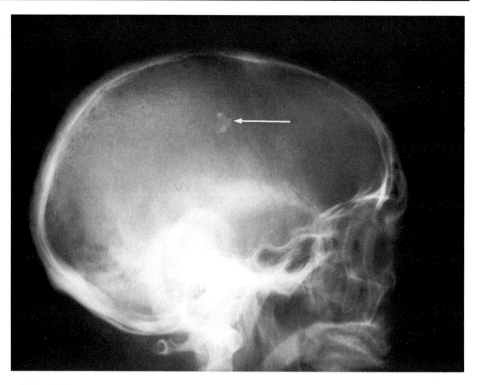

Fig. 3.22a   Lateral view showing intracerebral calcification (arrow) similar on this view to falx calcification.

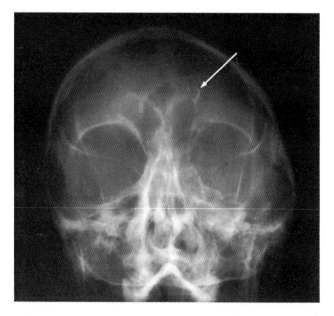

Fig. 3.22b   On the occipitofrontal view, the calcification is well on the left of the midline and therefore intracerebral.

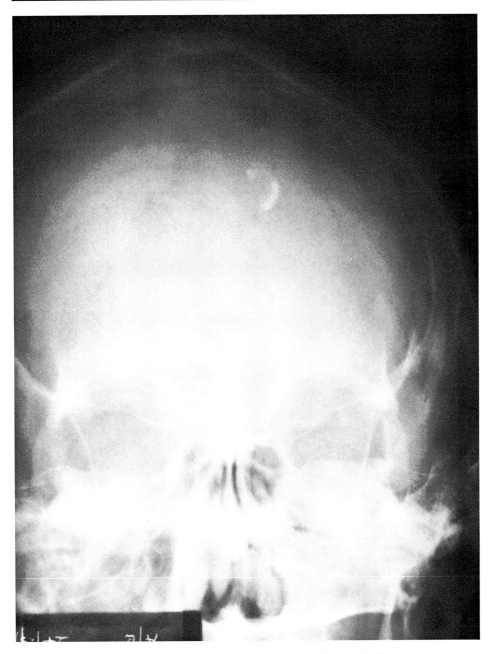

Fig. 3.22c   Close-up view of the intracerebral calcification.

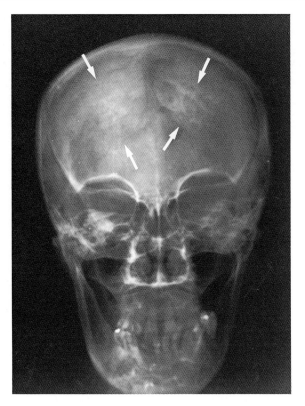

Fig. 3.23a Multiple line shadows in the frontal region but not crossing the midline, appearances typical of frontal hyperostosis.

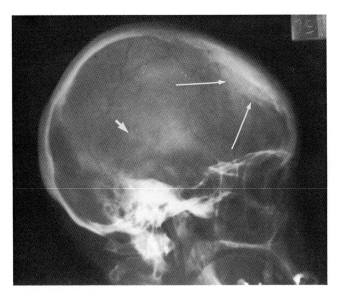

Fig. 3.23b Lateral view confirming the hyperostosis frontalis (long arrows). Calcified choroid plexus noted (arrow).

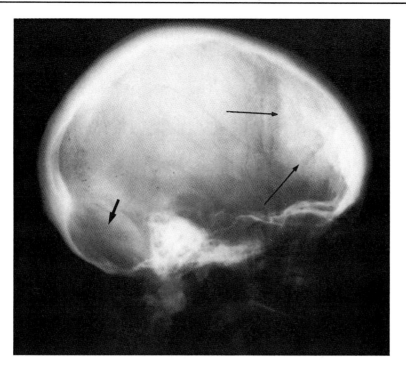

Fig. 3.24 Frontal hyperostosis (long arrows) but there is also marked thinning of the occipital bone (short arrow), often the first indication of Paget's disease (osteoporosis circumscripta cranialis).

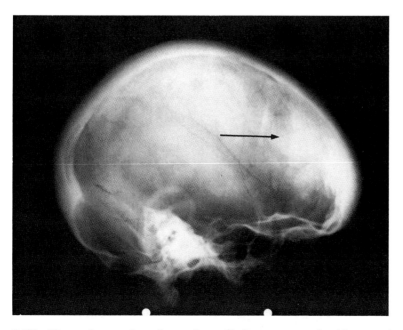

Fig. 3.25 Normal vascular channels well demonstrated with associated hyperostosis frontalis (arrow). Basal osteoporosis circumscripta cranialis of Paget's disease also present.

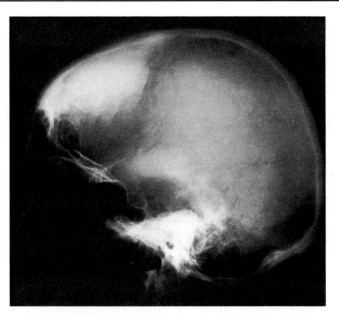

Fig. 3.26a   Marked increased bone density in the frontal region due to frontal hyperostosis, a common variant in the elderly.

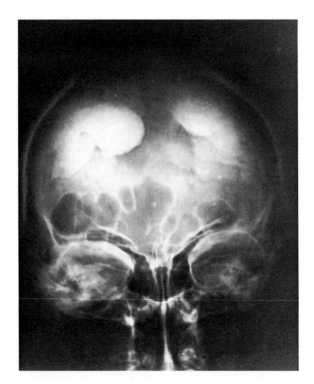

Fig. 3.26b   The bilateral sclerosis in both frontal regions, characteristic of hyperostosis frontalis, extremely marked in this case. Note how the central region remains unaffected even in a gross example. The large, multiloculated frontal sinus is a normal variant.

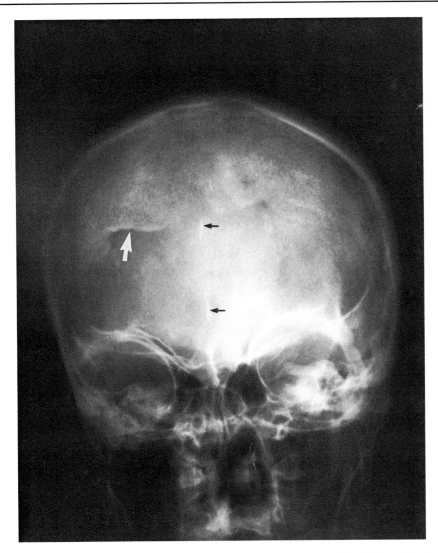

Fig. 3.27 Rotated occipitofrontal view showing calcified falx (black arrows) and lines of hyperostosis frontalis, a common variant in the elderly (white arrow), apparently more marked on the right owing to rotation.

Chapter 4

Linear fractures of the vault

The majority of vault factures are linear, caused by deceleration injuries when the head hits a flat surface, and are particularly common after road traffic accidents. The calvarium is forced inwards at the site of impact with simultaneous outbending at the periphery. If no fracture occurs with the inbending at the site of impact, the skull rebounds to its original form but the peripheral outbending may be sufficiently marked to cause a linear fracture that extends radially, both toward the region of impact and in the opposite direction (Gurdjian et al., 1953).

Minor fractures in the vast majority of cases are readily recognizable but when less obvious must be distinguished from vascular impression and channels, particularly in the temporoparietal region. However, linear fractures are usually seen as black straight lines with sharp edges and crossing vascular channels. It is usually the darkest long line seen on the radiograph and more radiolucent than vascular channels because fractures involve both tables of the skull (Figs. 4.1–4.5).

When the fracture changes direction, the track of the fracture does so abruptly, forming a well-defined obtuse angle; associated diastasis of a suture can occur if it runs into a suture line. Sutural diastasis is often more difficult to detect. Isolated sutural diastasis occurs more commonly in children and young adults before complete closure. Normally sutures are less than 1 mm in width and should not exceed 2 mm but the width of normal sutures shows considerable variation, frequently making the diagnosis of suture diastasis difficult (Fig. 4.6). However, it should be suspected when the margins of a suture are well defined and its width is equal to or greater than 2 mm, especially if unilateral (Figs. 4.7, 4.8). A diastatic fracture can be associated with a meningeal tear, and severe underlying local cerebral injury, resulting in ventricular enlargement or porencephaly. A porencephalic cavity resulting from traumatic cerebral infarction or haemorrhage can transmit cerebrospinal fluid (CSF) pulsations to the fracture, enlarging subsequently to produce a marked cranial defect (Lende, 1974).

A sharply defined fracture slowly loses its sharp borders and appears to widen slightly weeks to months after the original injury. If, however, disruption of the meninges at the fracture site occurs the arachnoid may herniate through the dura and become anchored in the fracture. Complex adhesions form and a leptomeningeal cyst may result, widening the fracture line and causing a large localized bone defect (Hillman et al., 1975).

Healing occurs slowly in adults, often over a period of two to three years, and the fracture finally disappears. During healing, new bone formation may bridge the fracture at various points, producing a discontinuous, inhomogeneous line. Alternatively, complete bone healing may not occur but, instead, fibrous tissue bridges the bone defect and the fracture line remains visible.

Rarely a fracture results in a traumatic arteriovenous fistula, with enlarging vascular grooves, as shown on serial skull films.

VASCULAR CHANNELS

Vascular channels may mimic skull fractures, appearing as linear transradiances, by producing bony grooves on the outer and inner tables, caused by branches of the external carotid artery, and are the main difficulty in diagnosing skull fractures. They are usually less lucent than fracture lines of the same size, frequently have sclerotic borders and wider tracks and often branch, becoming narrower distally.

Inner table of skull

The middle meningeal vessels

The middle meningeal artery (Fig. 4.6a) originates as a branch of the maxillary artery of the external carotid and is accompanied by veins draining into the pterygoid venous plexus. The middle meningeal artery enters the skull base through the foramen spinosum, grooving the anterior aspect of the squamous temporal bone, and divides into frontal and parietal branches. The frontal branch initially runs forwards towards the pterion and then curves backwards to form the anterior groove in the parietal bone, while the parietal branch runs backwards, well below the frontal branch, towards the posterior aspect of the parietal bone.

The grooves formed by the branches of the middle meningeal vessels are fortunately remarkably constant in position and their grooves on the inner table of the skull form relatively straight lines that otherwise could be interpreted as fractures. Furthermore the grooves on the temporal squama can be very radiolucent as this part of the bone is quite thin, particularly along the course of the parietal branch. The straight diagonal line often produced by this groove can easily be misinterpreted as a fracture. The sclerotic margin associated with vascular grooves is a most helpful discriminating feature.

The recognition of the meningeal grooves is equally important in somewhat different circumstances. The site and direction of parietal fractures must be carefully noted as to whether it crosses meningeal grooves, as a warning of the possibility of an extradural haematoma (Figs. 4.9, 4.10). In these circumstances, close observation and a neurological opinion is indicated.

Outer table of skull

The middle temporal arteries

The middle temporal artery, a branch of the superficial temporal artery, originates from the external carotid above the zygomatic arch, and perforates the temporal fascia where it gives branches to the temporalis muscles grooving the squamous part of the temporal bone.

The anterior and posterior branches of the deep temporal arteries

These branches (Figs. 4.1, 4.6a) originate from the internal maxillary artery within the infratemporal fossa, between the temporalis muscle and the outer table of the skull. The posterior branch runs along the anterior aspect of the temporal squama and the anterior branch along the lateral margin of the greater wing of sphenoid where it often grooves the outer table of the skull.

The supraorbital branch

The ophthalmic artery, after arising from the internal carotid at the carotid siphon, gives off its supraorbital branch that emerges through the supraorbital notch, then runs superiorly towards the coronal suture. The groove of the supraorbital artery tends to resemble a fracture of the frontal bone but can be identified when it is traced to its origin at the supraobital notch.

While in the vast majority of cases arterial grooves can be readily distinguished from fractures, it is particularly in the frontal and squamous temporal region that vascular channels often mimic fracture lines.

Diploic venous channels

Venous channels in the diploic space less frequently cause confusion, are predominantly in the frontal and parietal regions and tend to be multiple, wider and more tortuous than fractures, typically communicating with venous lakes (Figs. 4.11, 4.12, 4.13). Rarely, they may be sharply defined and straight, resembling a stellate type of fracture, particularly in the frontal bone on the lateral view, but branching channels are invariably present (Fig. 4.14). Additional views, whether frontal or tangential, will occasionally be required to resolve the difficulty.

CONCLUSION

Enlarged vascular grooves, particularly those caused by arteries, can provide important diagnostic information in cases of intracranial tumours such as meningiomas or angiomatous vascular malformations. However, venous channels can normally be very wide and without other signs do not signify intracranial pathology. Arterial grooves, particularly of the petrous temporal bone and in the frontal region, can mimic fractures, and fracture lines crossing the middle meningeal grooves can be of the utmost clinical significance. A clear understanding of the anatomy of the vascular channels is therefore essential in the interpretation of skull radiographs, particularly in the diagnosis of skull fractures where knowledge of the normal appearance is paramount (Fig. 4.15).

REFERENCES

Gurdjian E. S., Webster J. E., Lissner H. R. (1953). Observations on prediction of fracture site in head trauma. *Radiology*, **60**, 226.
Hillman R. S. L., Kieffer S. A., Oritz H., et al. (1975). Intraosseous leptomeningeal cysts of the posterior cranial fossa. *Radiology*, **116**, 655.
Lende R. A. (1974). Enlarging skull fractures of childhood. *Neuroradiology*, **7**, 119.

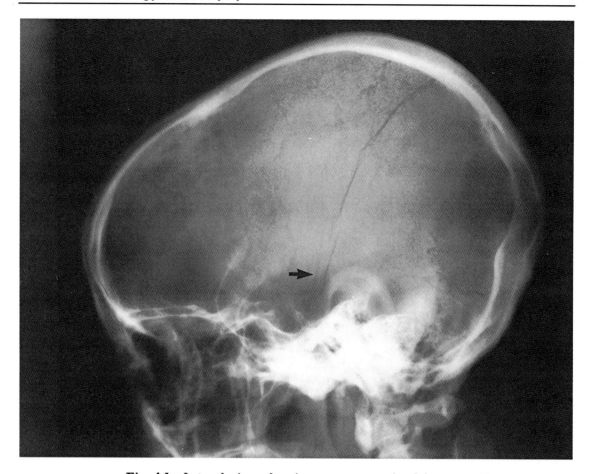

Fig. 4.1 Lateral view showing temporoparietal fracture. Note that the fracture line is darker and thinner than the vascular marking (superficial temporal vessels) lying just in front of the fracture, which is fainter but also straight and quite sharp (arrow). However, it ends in a small branching pattern. Note however the fracture line continues towards the base of the skull. Should there be symptoms or signs of petrous temporal involvement, CT of the skull base will be required to delineate the basal extension of the fracture.

Above right:
Fig. 4.2 A linear fracture of the temporal squama descends onto the skull base just posterior to the clivus. If indicated clinically, CT or a basal view would define the basal fracture.

Below right:
Fig. 4.3 Lateral view: there is a fracture in the right frontoparietal region showing as a dark black line which tapers inferiorly to end at the squamous temporal bone, crossing frontal venous channels. Note characteristic appearance of 'static' artefacts over the posterior parietal region (arrow). There should be no difficulty in their recognition. This artefact is caused by friction on the film prior to processing.

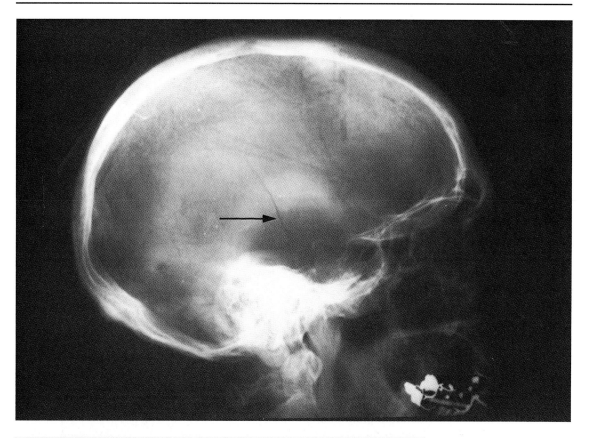

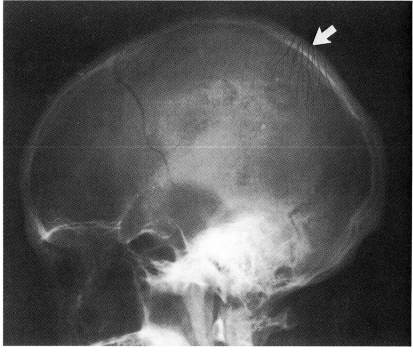

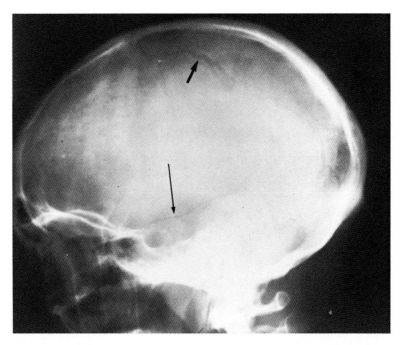

Fig. 4.4 Lateral view: fracture of the squamous temporal bone (long arrow) extending into the skull base in the region of the orbital plate. Large groove of a venous channel in the parietal region (bold arrow).

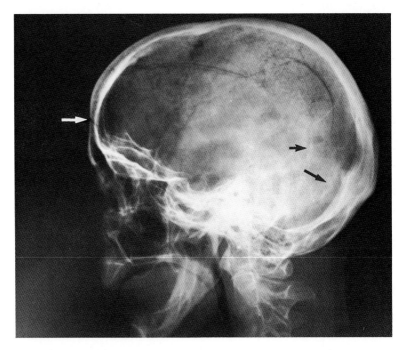

Fig. 4.5 An extensive frontoparietal linear fracture from just above the frontal sinuses (white arrow) to the posterior parietal region. White lines due to blood in the hair are seen posteriorly (black arrows).

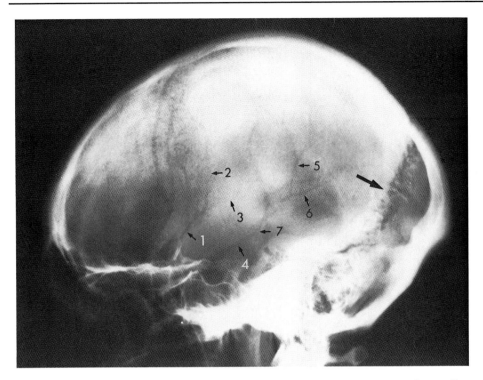

Fig. 4.6a Prominent vascular pattern due to venous channels well demonstrated on this view. The width of the lambdoid suture (large arrow) in its widest part measures only 1 mm, indicating a normal but prominent suture line.

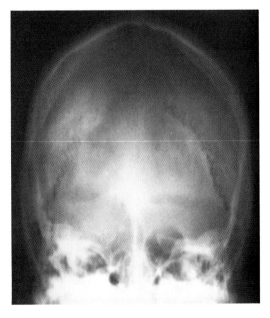

Meningeal artery grooves:
1. Frontal branch
2. Anterior division of the frontal branch
3. Posterior division of the frontal branch
4. Parietal branch
5. Superior division of the parietal branch
6. Inferior division of the parietal branch
7. Superficial temporal artery groove

Fig. 4.6b   Towne's view confirms this as a normal variant of the occipital suture and not sutural diastasis.

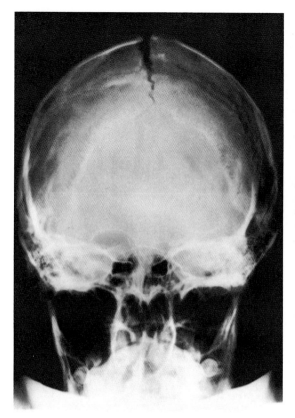

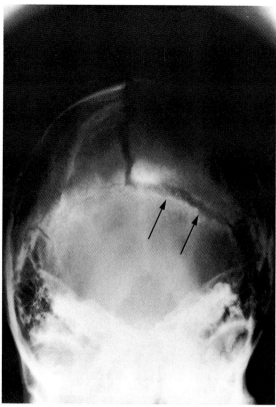

Fig. 4.7a This patient jumped off an express train sustaining sutural diastasis of the sagittal suture. In true sutural diastasis separation of the sutures is greater than 2 mm.

Fig. 4.7b Towne's view of the same patient showing the sagittal diastasis extending into the left parietooccipital suture (arrows). The abnormality is obvious when the two sides are compared.

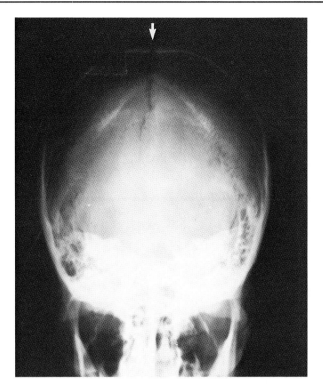

Fig. 4.8 Marked diastasis of the sagittal suture due to trauma seen on a Towne's view. Suture diastasis is equivalent to fracture.

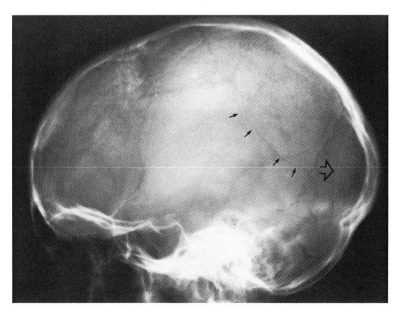

Fig. 4.9 Thin fracture line in posterior parietal region (small arrows) crossing vascular grooves as well as showing an extensive vascular pattern. Note the white line across the occiput (open arrow) caused by a cushion on which the head was resting.

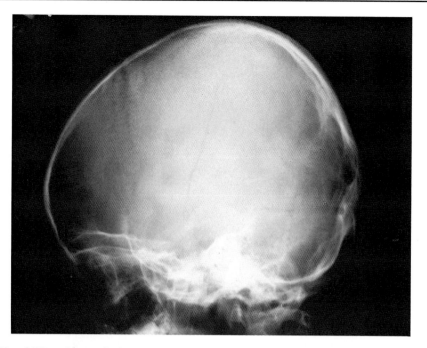

Fig. 4.10a   Lateral view of skull of a four-year-old girl showing a long-itudinal fracture in line with the pituitary fossa extending from the vertex down to the base.

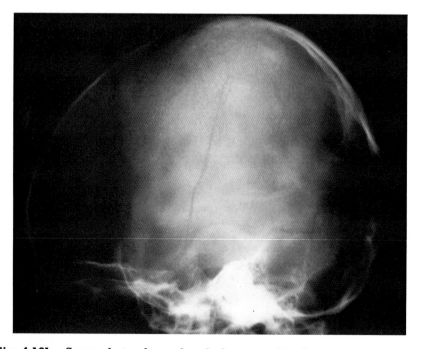

Fig. 4.10b   Somewhat enlarged and photographically enhanced print to demonstrate the fracture more clearly.

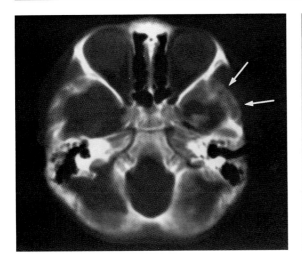

Fig. 4.10c Computed tomography scan of base of skull showing two fracture lines through the outer wall of the middle fossa (arrows).

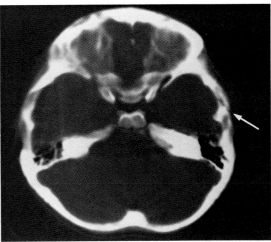

Fig. 4.10d The fracture line of the temporal bone shown on a CT section 1 cm higher (arrow).

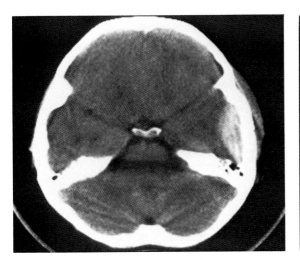

Fig. 4.10e A CT section 1 cm higher than Fig. 4.10d demonstrates an extradural haematoma as a lenticular high-attenuation area, as well as the scalp haematoma.

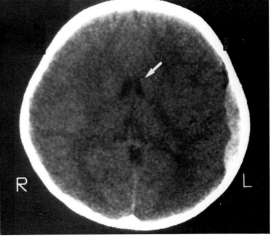

Fig. 4.10f A CT section through the anterior horns of the lateral ventricles showing slight midline shift (arrow) associated with the extradural haematoma.

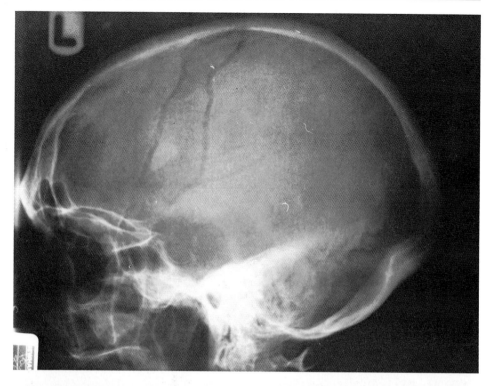

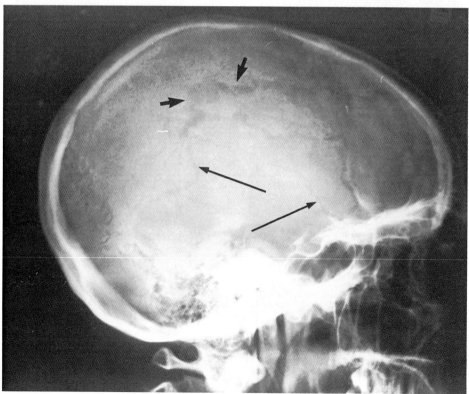

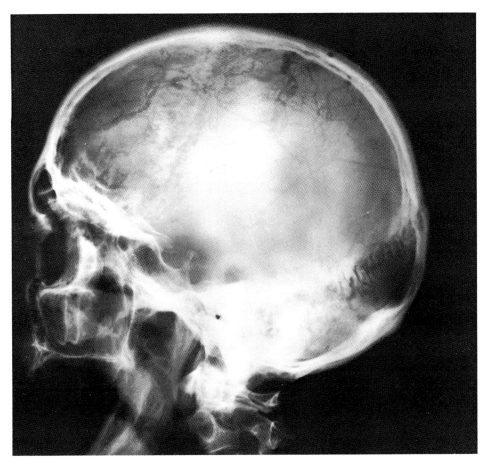

Fig. 4.13   Large frontal and parietal venous channels are shown, a not uncommon normal variant, particularly in the elderly.

Above left:
Fig. 4.11   Lateral view: note prominent venous channels at the bregmatic suture line. The channels are wide; this is a common anatomical site for a common normal variant.

Below left:
Fig. 4.12   Lateral view: venous channels (long arrows) are well demonstrated on this view. They tend to be wide and more tortuous than fractures and typically communicate with venous lakes (short arrows). The common sites of these channels are in the frontal and parietal regions.

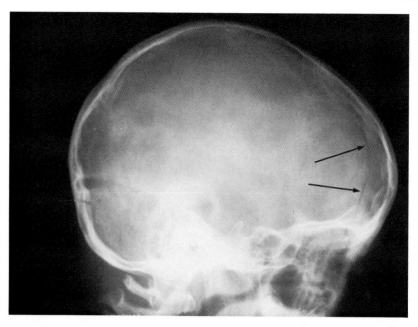

Fig. 4.14a   Lateral view showing a fracture (arrows) in the frontal bone. The fracture line is blacker with sharper margins and much more regular and less branching than the venous lakes (see Fig. 4.12).

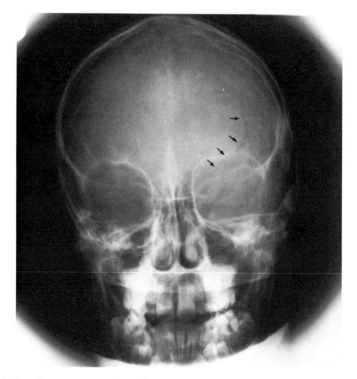

Fig. 4.14b   Anteroposterior view confirms the fracture of the left frontal bone (arrows).

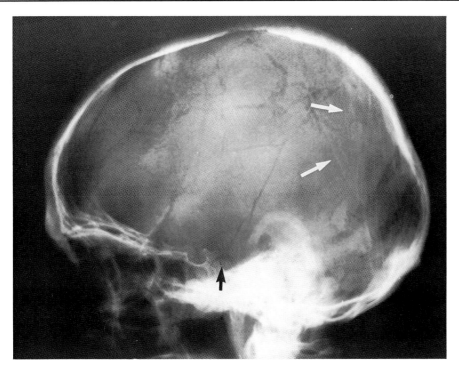

Fig. 4.15a   Lateral view showing a fracture in the parietal region extending through the squamous temporal bone, onto the base of the skull. There is a fluid level in the sphenoidal sinus (Fig. 4.15b) indicating that the fracture extends onto the base of the middle fossa and in addition a small crescent of subdural air (black arrow) is shown. Note also the streaky white lines (white arrows) over the occipital region due to blood in the hair and prominent venous channels in the parietal bone. This case illustrates the care required in viewing and interpreting skull radiographs.

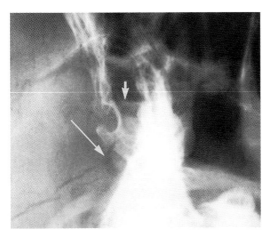

Fig. 4.15b   Enlarged view showing the vertical fracture through the temporal squama extending onto the base and the sickle of subarachnoid air (long arrow) as well as the fluid level in the sphenoidal sinus (short arrow).

Chapter 5

Depressed fractures of the vault

A depressed fracture by definition is more likely to be associated with underlying dural or cerebral injury. The force producing a depressed fracture is concentrated in a small area and arises from trauma by hammers or similar weapons; the bone depression can usually be palpated. The greater force needed to produce a depressed fracture results in inbending of the cranium with fragmentation, and multiple radial fractures extending out from the depressed fragment. In adults the blow is often of sufficient force to drive both tables of the skull inwards, producing a compound fracture (Figs. 5.1, 5.2) which is therefore almost always associated with overlying soft-tissue laceration. Of even greater importance, there may be a tear of the dura mater covering the brain and cerebral contusion or laceration.

Characteristically the fracture of the inner table is more extensive than that of the outer table and bone fragments become displaced under the intact skull (Fig. 5.3). Indriven fragments tend to spring back towards the surface, leaving damaged tissue and sometimes foreign material deeper in the brain than might be expected from examination of the radiographs.

Clearly, dural tears provide a portal for infection, but if the tear extends into the sagittal sinus or one of the transverse sinuses torrential haemorrhage either at the time of injury or during a subsequent operation can occur. Furthermore an intracerebral haematoma can complicate a cerebral laceration caused by a penetrating bone fragment (Figs. 5.4–5.6).

Guthkelch (1960) drew attention to a small but important group of patients in whom a sharp object enters the skull through the orbital roof leaving only a small cut in the skin. Such objects include knitting needles, umbrella tips, swords, indoor television aerials, screw drivers, ball-point pens, toys and even a stiletto heel. In these injuries deep penetration often goes unrecognized and the development of an intracranial haematoma or meningitis may be the first evidence of a serious injury. The faintest trace of periorbital gas may be the only clue apart from a possible opaque foreign body.

More than 50% of patients with depressed fractures do not lose consciousness (Gordon, 1974). Costly mistakes can be avoided if a depressed fracture is suspected in every patient with a scalp laceration. Probing of the wound, or palpation of the skull by the tip of the index finger is the most reliable way to make the diagnosis.

Haemorrhage under the scalp gives rise to a deceptive swelling sometimes called a 'doughnut haematoma'. The periphery of the swelling presents a firm, raised margin; the softer centre appears to be more deeply placed, giving the false impression of a depressed fracture. Careful palpation will usually lead to the correct diagnosis.

The radiographic signs may be obvious, usually on the tangential view, but can be quite subtle on the *en-face* view showing the fracture when only a faint irregular ring with radiating lines may be seen, or a subtle white line when the fracture only involves a single piece of bone without being significantly comminuted (Fig. 5.7). In the parasagittal region, as well as the temporal region, depressed fractures are particularly difficult to detect because the surrounding bones are dense and may obscure the fracture.

Tangential views are extremely helpful in delineating the extent of the injury and in showing how far the bone has been driven inwards. If the area affected is large, the normal contour of the vault is lost, and the cranium is flattened, becoming asymmetrical (Fig. 5.8). If the depression is small, the white lines representing the inner and outer tables of the fragment appear discontinuous with the rest of the vault and often sharply delineated (Figs. 5.9, 5.10).

Patients with depressed skull fracture will require neurosurgical intervention, hence referral to a specialist centre is mandatory, where early CT scanning will be performed.

Note that blood in the hair appearing as white lines can mimic a depressed fracture, particularly on the lateral view (Figs. 5.11, 5.12). There will however be no evidence of depression on the tangential view and no clinical evidence of a depressed fracture.

REFERENCES

Gordon G. S. (1974). Depressed fractures and missile wounds of the skull. *Br. J. Hosp. Med.*, **August**, 177.

Guthkelch A. N. (1960). Apparently trivial wounds of the eyelids with intracranial damage. *Br. Med. J.*, **ii**, 842.

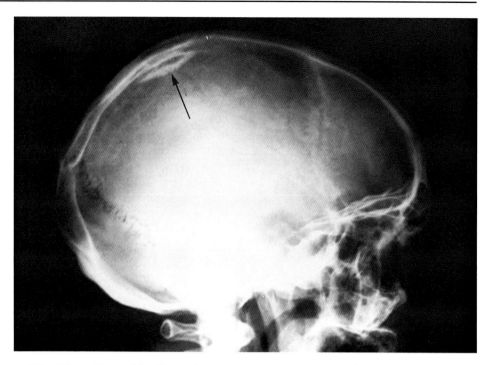

Fig. 5.1a   The white line of a depressed fracture (arrow) is quite thick in this case and associated fracture lines are not visible.

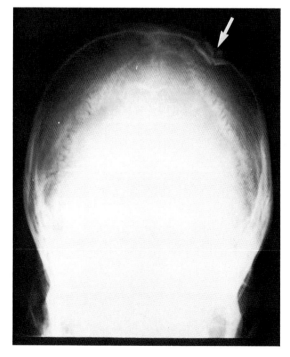

Fig. 5.1b   On the Towne's view the depression (arrow) is clearly visible together with the central fracture.

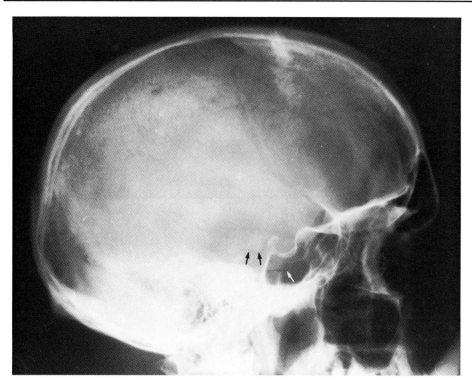

Fig. 5.2a   There is only a vague suggestion of an opacity projected just posterior to the clivus (black arrows) in a patient with trauma to the side of the head. Note the visible fracture line projected over the sphenoid sinus (white arrow).

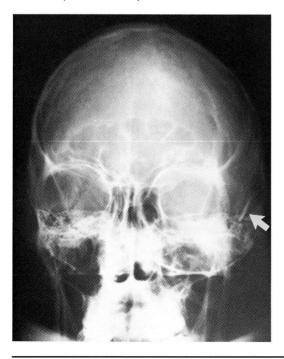

Fig. 5.2b   The frontal, tangential view shows the white line of a depressed fracture of the temporal bone (arrow), only faintly shown as a density posterior to the sella turcica in Fig. 5.2a.

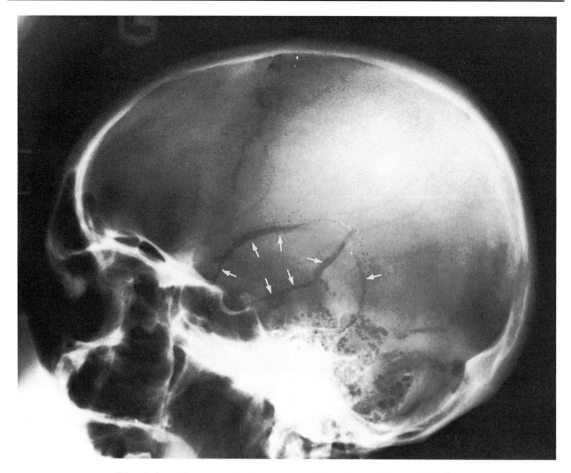

Fig. 5.3a   A severely depressed fracture of the right temporal bone in a patient who was mugged and beaten on the head with a hammer. Note the circular fracture line indicating a depressed fracture (arrows).

Above right:
Fig. 5.3b   The marked depression of the fracture (arrow) is well demonstrated on the tangential view, with increased density of the depressed bone fragment.

Below right:
Fig. 5.3c   In CT sections above the level of the fracture, the subaponeurotic haematoma is demonstrated (white arrows) but there is also intracerebral haemorrhage (black arrow), swelling of the frontal lobe and slight compression and displacement of the frontal pole of the lateral ventricle.

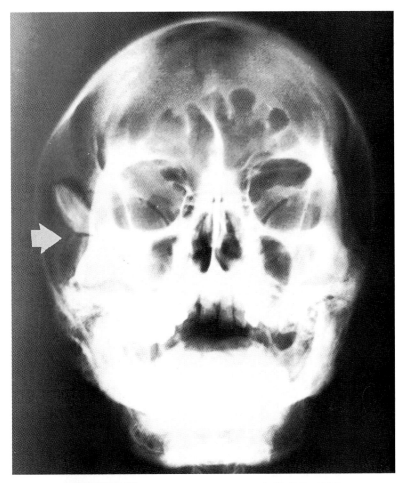

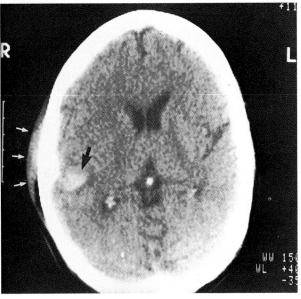

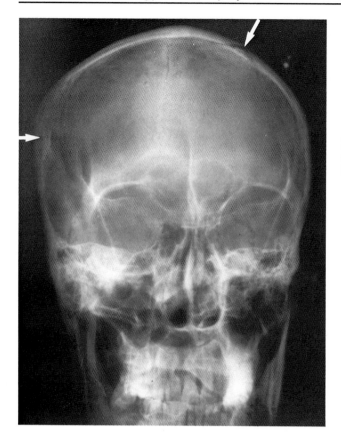

Fig. 5.4a Frontal view showing a right depressed parietal fracture and a left frontal stellate fracture (arrows).

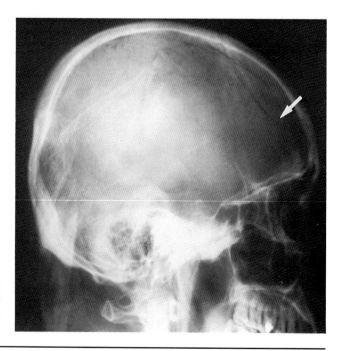

Fig. 5.4b The parietal and frontal fractures overlap on the lateral view with the frontal fracture (arrow) extending towards the base.

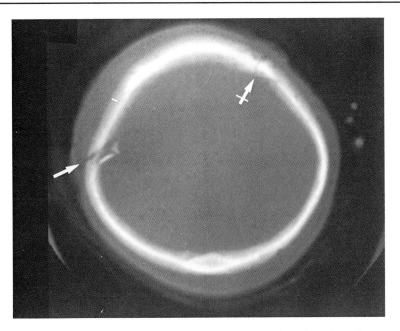

Fig. 5.5a Axial CT section towards the vertex showing the depressed bone fragments driven into the cortex of the cerebrum beneath the linear fracture (arrow). A large subaponeurotic haematoma is also present with a smaller haematoma over the left frontal linear fracture (crossed arrow).

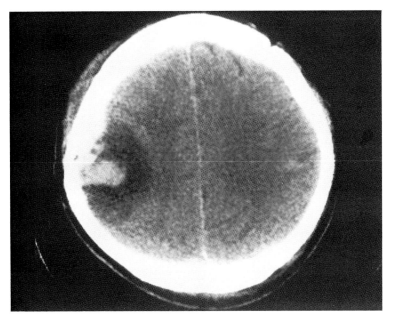

Fig. 5.5b Soft-tissue setting at a slightly lower level showing a high-attenuation lesion due to intracerebral haemorrhage with surrounding low-attenuation oedema. The extracranial haematoma is also visible.

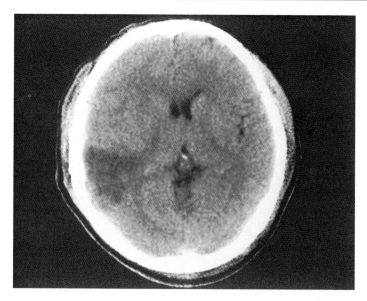

Fig. 5.6   At a lower level the mass effect is shown by the compression of the right frontal horn, displacement of the midline to the left and effacement of the cortical sulci on the right.

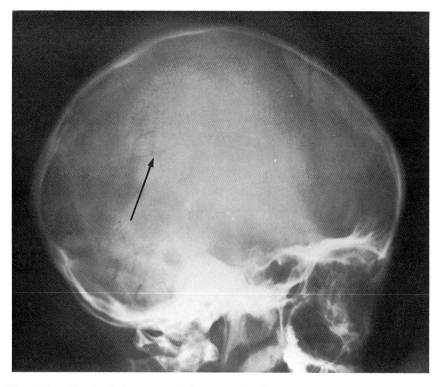

Fig. 5.7a   Typical depressed fracture in the posterior parietal region with lines radiating from the centre (arrow) and a circumlinear fracture line at the periphery.

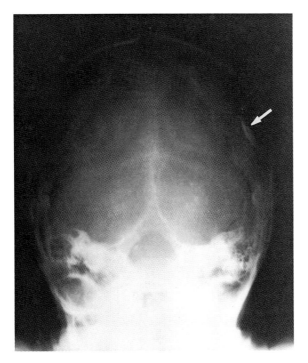

Fig. 5.7b   Towne's view: the depressed fracture (arrow) is even more obvious on this projection.

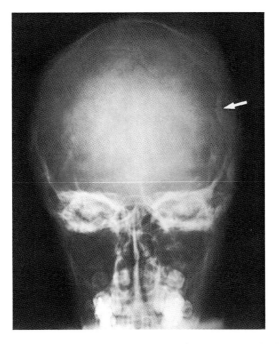

Fig. 5.7c   On the frontal view the depression (arrow) is demonstrated with the bone fragments appearing dense by being tilted into the line of the x-ray beam.

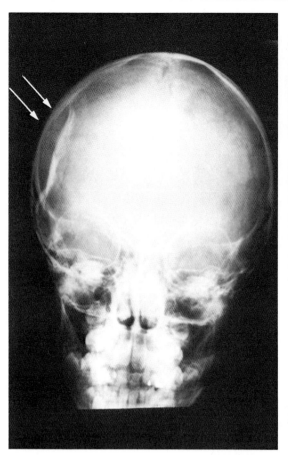 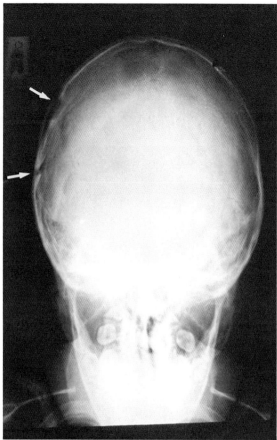

Fig. 5.8a   Extensive depression over the right temporal region (arrows).

Fig. 5.8b   Comminuted fracture (arrows) of the right parietal bone with slight depression seen on a Towne's view.

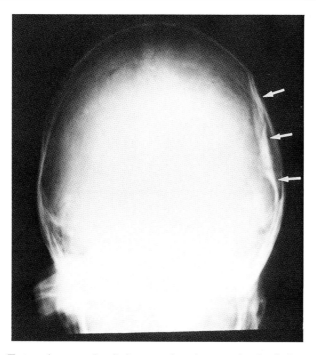

Fig. 5.8c Extensive marked depression (arrows) of a left parietal fracture on a Towne's view.

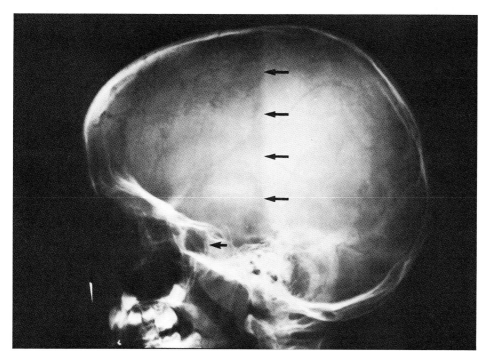

Fig. 5.8d The extent of the injury is well demonstrated on this view. There is a large collection of air within the cranium (long arrows) together with fluid in the sphenoidal sinus (short arrow).

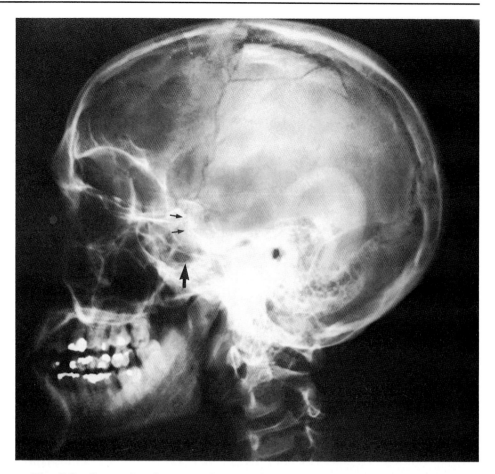

Fig. 5.9 Severely depressed comminuted fractures of the parietal region. The anterior vertical fracture extends onto the skull base (arrows). There is a fluid level in the sphenoidal sinus confirming a basal fracture. The film was taken with the patient sitting.

Top right:
Fig. 5.10a Lateral view showing an extensive fracture around the pterion (white arrows). Note that the white lines (black arrows) at the end of the curvilinear fracture are suggestive of a depressed fracture.

Lower left:
Fig. 5.10b This Towne's view shows the extent of the fracture (arrow) but the depression is not demonstrated.

Lower right:
Fig. 5.10c Frontal view showing the extent of depression (arrows) in this particular fracture.

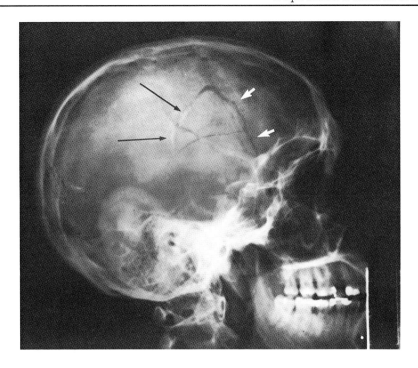

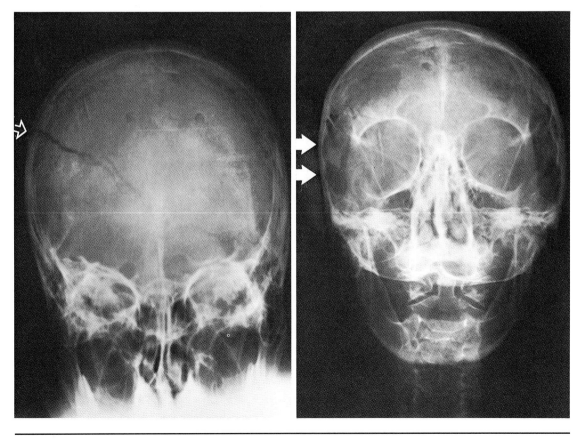

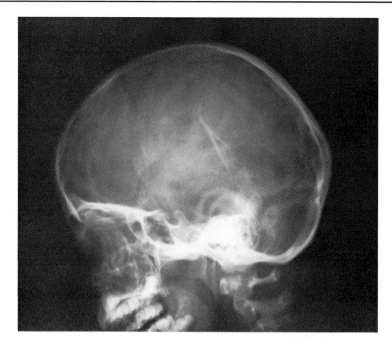

Fig. 5.11   On the lateral view the white lines due to blood in the hair are even more obvious and could easily be mistaken for a 'white line' fracture.

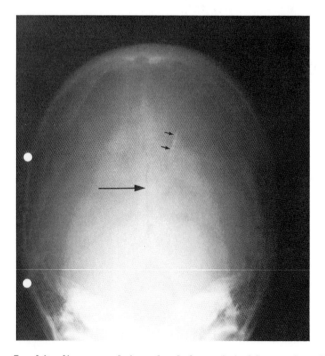

Fig. 5.12   A white line overlying the left occipital bone (small arrows) was caused by blood in the hair and not a depressed fracture. The central vertical transradiant line (large arrow) is due to a metopic suture and not a fracture.

Chapter 6

Fractures in children

In children, there is a higher incidence of fractures in skull radiographs taken for trauma than in adults. Three reports, totalling 6035 skull examinations revealed 1957 skull fractures (Hall, 1979). If the adult criteria (e.g. Bell and Loop, 1971) in selecting patients for skull radiographs had been applied to children, a high proportion would have been missed, possibly as high as 35% (Desmet et al., 1979). In Desmet's series, six such 'missed' fractures had an uneventful outcome. He and other workers (Desmet et al., 1979; Harwood-Nash et al., 1971; Roberts and Shopfer, 1972; Boulis et al., 1978) concluded that the presence or absence of a fracture in a child neither correlated with the clinical findings nor affected management. Nevertheless the development of a leptomeningeal cyst as a complication of a skull fracture in children is well recognized and failure of healing of the fracture on the skull film is an early sign of this complication.

Quite clearly, clinical judgement is all important in deciding which child should have a radiographic examination of the skull for head injury. However, in this country all children with skull fractures are admitted to hospital for observation and in this way skull radiographs affect management. At present, we recommend skull radiography for trauma in children below the age of three years.

RADIOLOGICAL ANATOMY

In infants, the calvarium is relatively large compared to the face and base of the skull. At birth the head-to-face ratio is approximately 4:1 (Figs. 6.1–6.10), in adults the ratio is 3:2. The bones are still incompletely mineralized and separated from each other by radiolucent sutures and fontanelles (Figs. 6.11, 6.12). A knowledge of the normal sutural anatomy of the skull is essential for an accurate reading of the radiographs.

The metopic suture

The frontal bone is divided into two by the midline frontal or metopic suture, being completely obliterated in the vast majority by the third year, but persists in 10% throughout life. This is known as cranium bifidum occultum (Figs. 6.13, 6.14 and see Fig. 5.8).

The coronal, sagittal and lambdoid sutures persist into adult life. The width and visibility of the sutures vary markedly, particularly from ages four to eight years, and should not be mistaken for evidence of increased intracranial pressure; any perisutural sclerosis can further accentuate the suture lines.

The occipital sutures

The occipital bone is formed by four separate components surrounding the foramen magnum: the basiocciput anterior to the foramen magnum and articulating with the body of the sphenoid bone, the two lateral occipital portions on each side of the foramen magnum, and the squamous portion posteriorly. In addition, the superior (interparietal) portion of the occipital squama is usually formed from two separate ossification centres. The various components of the occipital bone prior to fusion are separated by transradiant cartilage but disappear by the third year, although the occipitomastoid suture may remain prominent and simulate a fracture.

Midline occipital fissure

A midline fissure is present inferiorly in the course of development of the supraoccipital portion of the occipital squama, closing by apposition of its lateral margins as well as by the descent of a midline (Kerkring's) process. If the midline process does not completely descend and the lateral margins of the fissure do not fuse, a persistent midline occipital fissure results but does not usually extend to within 2 cm of the foramen magnum; nevertheless, it can mimic a fracture.

Lateral fissures of the foramen magnum

Failure of fusion of Kerkring's process produces short lucent lines close to the midline from the posterior lip of the foramen magnum. While they are usually bilateral, a unilateral fissure may well be mistaken for a fracture.

Failure of fusion of the other components of the occipital bone results in well recognized normal variants. The persisting sutures include the transverse occipital suture between the interparietal and supraoccipital squama, the superior median fissure in the midline in the interparietal squama, the lateral interparietal sutures along the supralateral margin of the interparietal squama and the basioccipital suture. Fusion usually occurs by the third year. Failure of fusion of the basisphenoid with the basiocciput results in a marked defect particularly well shown on CT but also on the basal (submentovertical) view.

Lateral cranial sutures

As the anterior fontanelle begins to fuse, the appearances may suggest the presence of a depressed fracture on the lateral view. However, the diamond shape seen on the Towne's view is characteristic and readily distinguished from a fracture.

Lateral sphenoidal sutures

The greater wing of the sphenoid articulates laterally with the frontal, zygomatic, parietal and temporal bones and they meet at the pterion. On the lateral view they overlie the orbits, the body of the sphenoid and the floor of the frontal fossa. These suture lines may occasionally mimic a fracture.

Similarly the squamosal and mastoid sutures can occasionally simulate a fracture but their known positions and symmetry will help in their recognition (see Figs. 2.1b, 2.4a).

Parietal fissure

Parietal fissures can occur in neonates owing to persistent strips of membranous bone matrix; they disappear as the child matures, but can be mistaken for fractures. If persistent, this suture divides the parietal bone into upper and lower segments seen on lateral skull radiographs and if unilateral, the side of the head with the suture is often larger than the opposite side.

Wormian bones

Ectopic ossification centres are not uncommonly seen along the sutures and in fontanelles called wormian bones (Fig. 6.15 and see Fig. 7.17b). These are often multiple and found along the lambdoid and sagittal sutures. Though a normal variant, the presence of multiple wormian bones can be associated with osteogenesis imperfecta (Fig. 6.16), cleidocranial dysostosis and cretinism, among other conditions.

In infants the transradiancy caused by the junction of the frontal and ethmoid bones may simulate a transverse fracture through the two bones on the lateral view. The nasofrontal suture may persist into adult life and should also not be confused with a fracture.

RADIOGRAPHY

In children with skull trauma, a good lateral and occipitofrontal view should be adequate and should be taken as quickly as possible without upsetting the child, especially toddlers as it is almost impossible to hold a struggling child down for a satisfactory film (Fig. 6.17). In small babies, one should aim to take the films after a feed. Wrapping the child in a cover or giving it a feeding bottle are effective measures in settling the child.

As the child often moves during skull radiography, it may be necessary to repeat a film for a better view but it is worth remembering that one is giving the child another dose of radiation and while the film may not be ideal, should be accepted, provided it is diagnostic (Fig. 6.6).

For a child under six years of age, a lateral horizontal beam is not essential as the sphenoids are then not sufficiently aerated to show an air-fluid level (Figs. 6.5, 6.7). Similarly, the AP supine projection is easier and far more acceptable than the PA erect, being less likely to result in repeat films.

Recognition of birth trauma on radiographs may be difficult because moulding of the fetal head may produce depression of the calvarium and simulate a depressed fracture. However, overlapping of the parietal and occipital bones posteriorly is abnormal and does represent a fracture (Fig. 6.18).

There is usually no difficulty in distinguishing linear fractures in children (Figs. 6.19–6.21) from unfused sutures. Healing is quicker than in adults, the lesion usually disappearing in young in children four to six months after injury, but may take up to one year in older children. Because of the possibility of a leptomeningeal cyst, a follow-up radiograph should be taken at three months and if the fracture is still as obvious, repeated at six months (Fig. 6.22).

Although a depressed fracture (Figs. 6.23–6.27) is, as a rule, comminuted, the ping-pong fracture of infancy is the exception. Because of the softness and resilience of the infantile calvarium, inbending without a fracture line may occur and is best seen tangentially. In fact, the *en-face* views appear normal, but the slight increased density will be seen if the depression in the calvarium is projected tangentially.

In children, various hair styles may produce superimposed shadows that must not be confused with fractures or other pathology, particularly those due to intracranial calcifications (see Chapter 9).

REFERENCES AND FURTHER READING

Allen W. E., Kier E. L., Rothman S. L. G. (1973). Pitfalls in the evaluation of skull trauma. *Radiol. Clin. North Am.*, **11**, 479.

Bell R. S., Loop J. W. (1971). The utility and futility of radiographic skull examination for trauma. *New Engl. J. Med.*, **284**, 236.

Boulis Z. F., Dick R., Barnes N. R. (1978). Head injuries in children – aetiology, symptoms, physical findings and X-ray wastage. *Br. J. Radiol.*, **51**, 851.

Desmet A. A., Fryback D. G., Thornbury J. R. (1979). A second look at the utility of radiographic skull examination for trauma. *Am. J. Roentgenol.*, **132**, 95.

Gyll C., Blake N. (1986). *Paediatric Diagnostic Imaging*, pp. 94–103. London: Heinemann Medical.

Hall F. M. (1979). Radiological skull examination in trauma. *Am. J. Roentgenol.*, **132**, 1027.

Harwood-Nash D. C., Hendrick E. B., Hudson A. R. (1971). The significance of skull fractures in children. *Radiology*, **101**, 151.

Roberts F., Shopfer C. E. (1972). Plain skull roentgenograms in children with head trauma. *Am. J. Roentgenol.*, **114**, 230.

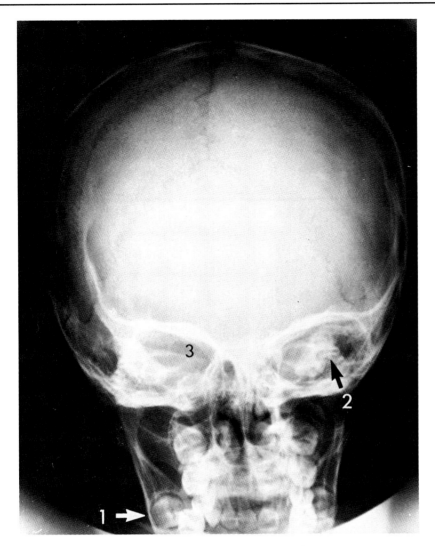

Fig. 6.1 Normal child, occipitofrontal view: the sutures are more obvious than in adults. Unerupted teeth (1) are visible and there is better definition of the middle ear, semicircular canals (2) and internal auditory meatuses (3) than in adults.

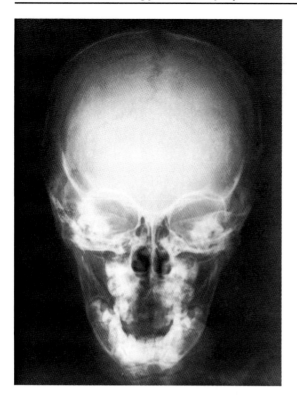

Fig. 6.2 Normal child, occipitofrontal view: the sutures are well demonstrated but no paranasal sinuses are visible.

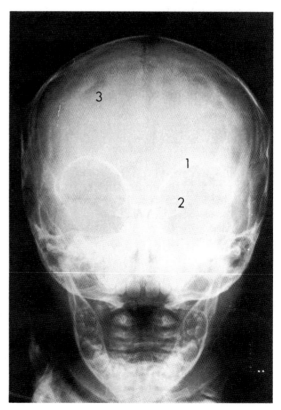

Fig. 6.3 Occipitofrontal projection of a normal child; the orbital margins (1) and lesser wing of the sphenoid (2) are prominent. The curved transradiances in the cranium are a common normal variant (3).

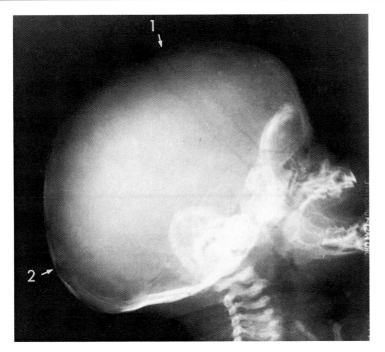

Fig. 6.4 An infant lateral skull film showing a normal open anterior fontanelle (1) and closed posterior fontanelle (2). The calvarial bones are thin and the inner and outer tables have, as yet, not been differentiated.

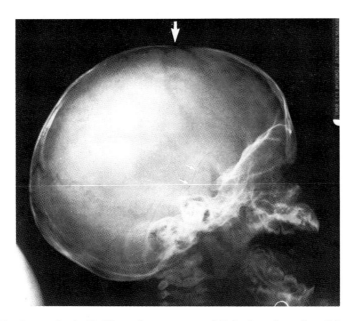

Fig. 6.5 Lateral skull film of a young child showing the thin normal transradiant line of the parietotemporal suture (small arrows). No air is, as yet, present in the sphenoidal sinus, but the inner and outer tables of the calvarium are becoming visible. The anterior fontanelle is still open (large arrow).

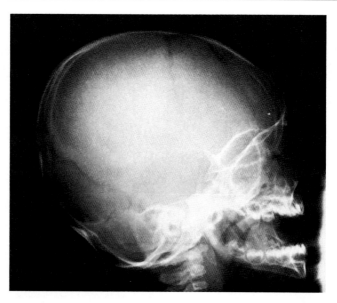

Fig. 6.6   The film is not truly lateral but nevertheless is quite diagnostic and therefore a repeat examination is unnecessary.

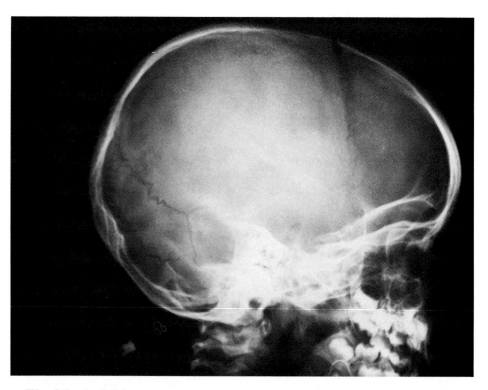

Fig. 6.7   In children sutures are even more prominent on the lateral view, particularly posteriorly (parietooccipital), but not the sphenoidal sinus as it does not aerate before the age of six years. Brow-up views for fluid levels are therefore not essential as in adults.

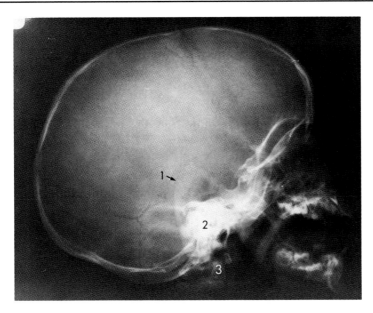

Fig. 6.8 Lateral view showing ear lobes (1), external auditory meatus (2) and odontoid peg (3). Note that the odontoid peg has not fused to the axis yet and note the forward position of the atlas in relation to the peg.

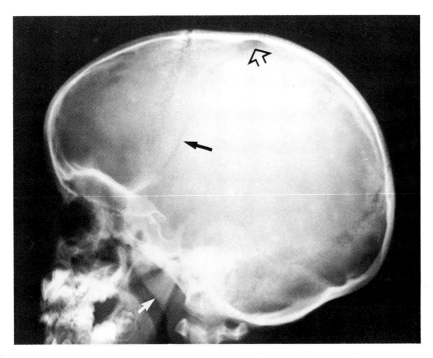

Fig. 6.9 Lateral view of a child's skull showing a prominent venous groove (black solid arrow) originating from a venous lake (open arrow). The adenoidal soft tissues are also well demonstrated (white arrow).

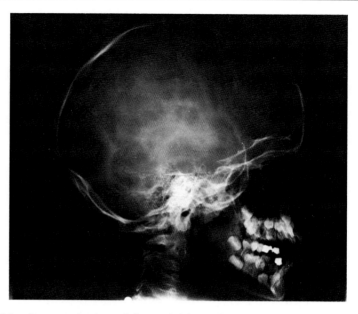

Fig. 6.10   An overexposed lateral view showing the appearance of a copper-beaten skull in the parietal region, a common normal variant.

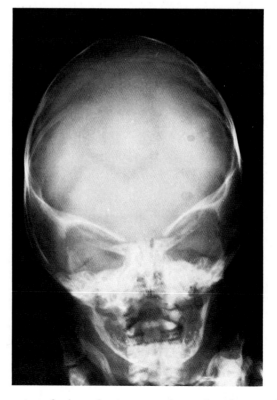

Fig. 6.11   Premature fusion of suture produces the abnormal shape of the skull with a markedly pointed cranium and increased bone density.

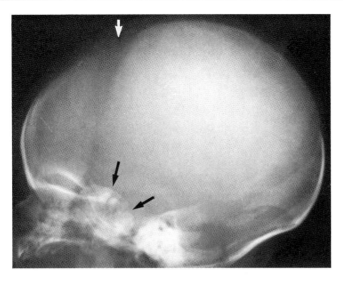

Fig. 6.12 Congenital small orbits owing to absent eyeballs associated with bone overgrowths around sella turcica. Note the wide frontoparietal suture of neonates with a widely open anterior fontanelle (white arrow), and marked bone sclerosis around the sella turcica (black arrows).

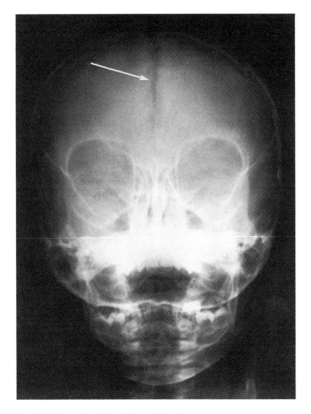

Fig. 6.13 A typical metopic suture is shown, a common normal variant in a child and particularly prominent in this case (arrow).

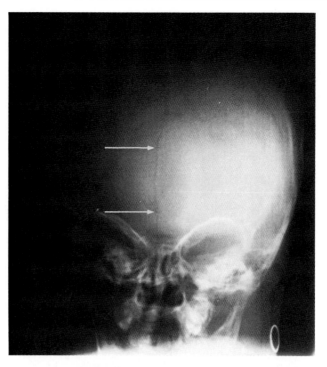

Fig. 6.14a   A long vertical linear fracture (arrows) of the occipital bone runs down to the skull base projected below the frontal bone, quite different to the metopic suture in the preceding illustration.

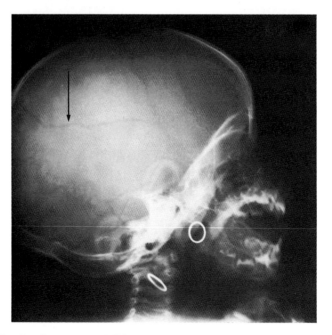

Fig. 6.14b   In the same child there was also a marked fracture of the parietal bone (arrow).

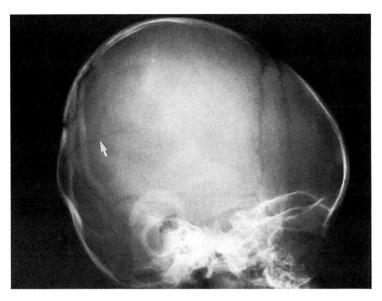

Fig. 6.15a There is a horizontal fracture of the occipital bone extending anteriorly (arrow).

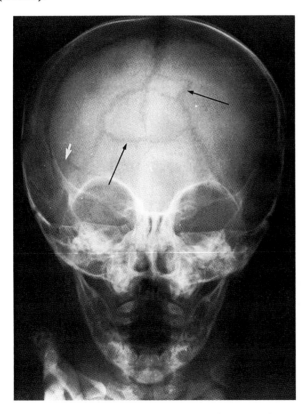

Fig. 6.15b The fracture is also shown on the frontal view as it extends into the parietal bone (white arrow). In addition the film shows wormian bone within the lambdoid suture (black arrows).

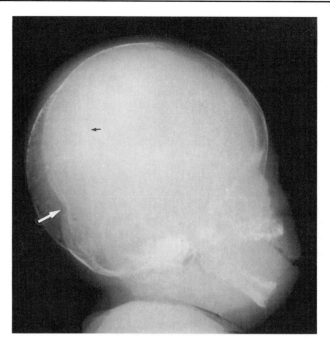

Fig. 6.16a   Very thin bone of a child with congenital osteogenesis imperfecta on a film showing a depressed fracture of the occipital bone (white arrow). There is also a straight line artefact due to superimposed sponge pads (black arrow).

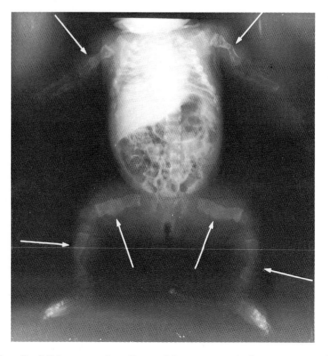

Fig. 6.16b   A child severely affected by congenital osteogenesis imperfecta with gross multiple fractures (arrows) of almost all her bones.

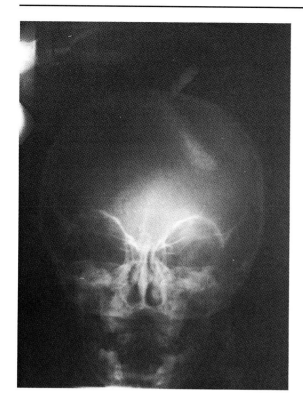

Fig. 6.17a Frontal view, overexposed and mother's fingers including ring indicate how not to hold the child's head.

Fig. 6.17b Lateral view, almost diagnostic of mother's hands but far too black to see the child's skull. Hopefully examinations such as these will not occur in your hospital.

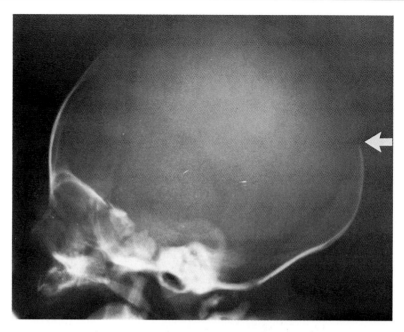

Fig. 6.18 Overriding of the occipitoparietal bones (arrow) following birth trauma from a forceps delivery.

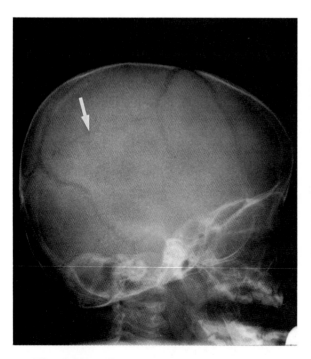

Fig. 6.19a The horizontal parietal fracture stretches between the prominent lambdoid and coronal sutures (arrow).

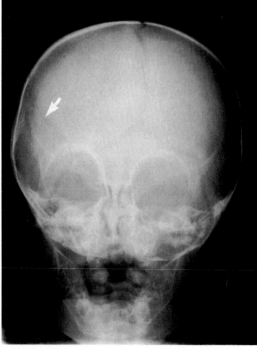

Fig. 6.19b Prominent sutures in a child's skull but also a fracture of the parietal bone (arrow).

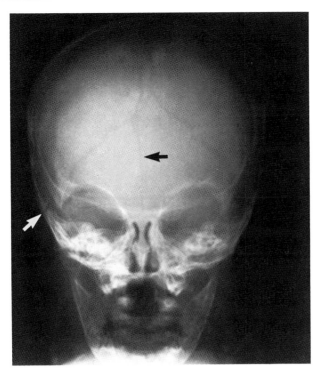

Fig. 6.20a   A child with extensive right-sided parietal and temporal fractures. The temporal fracture is well shown on the frontal view (white arrow). A metopic suture (black arrow) is also present.

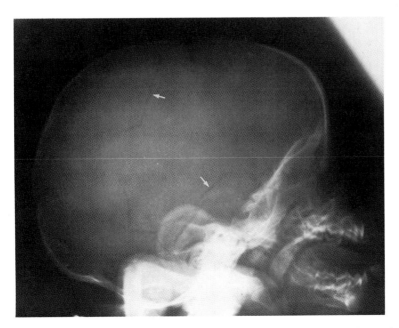

Fig. 6.20b   On the lateral view both the parietal and temporal linear fractures are well demonstrated (arrows).

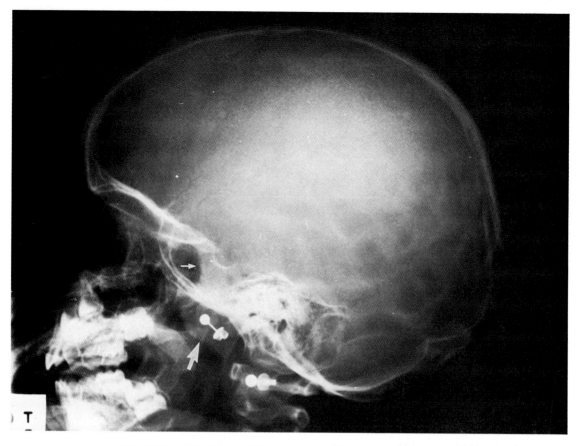

Fig. 6.21   A fluid level is present in the sphenoid sinus (small arrow) and there is prominence of the posterior nasopharynx soft tissues (large arrow) indicating the possibility of a basal fracture with the danger of subsequent meningitis.

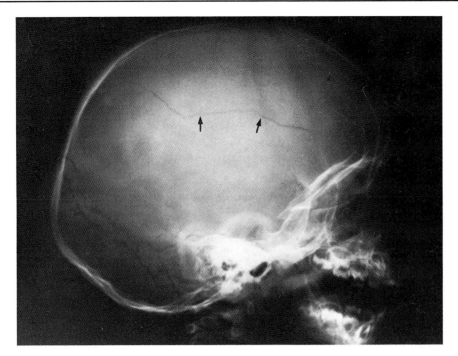

Fig. 6.22a   Lateral view of the skull showing an extensive horizontal parietal fracture (arrows).

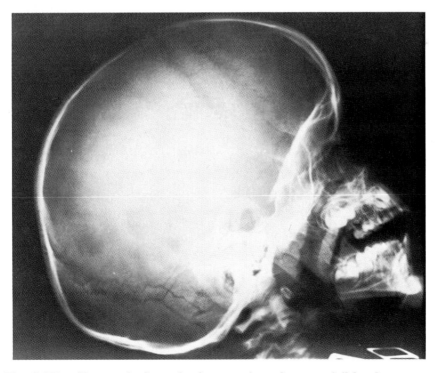

Fig. 6.22b   Six months later the fracture is no longer visible, the sutures however are well demonstrated.

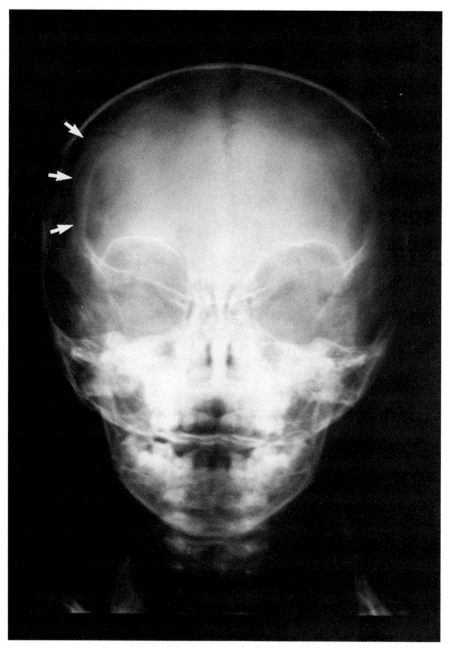

Fig. 6.23a   Extensive parietal fracture on the right (arrows) but no evidence to suggest depression of the adjacent zone.

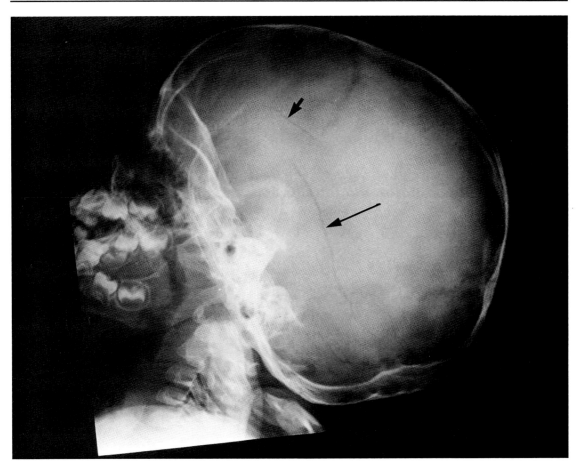

Fig. 6.23b   The lateral view shows the extensive linear parietal fracture (long arrow) and a smaller horizontal fracture of the frontal bone (short arrow).

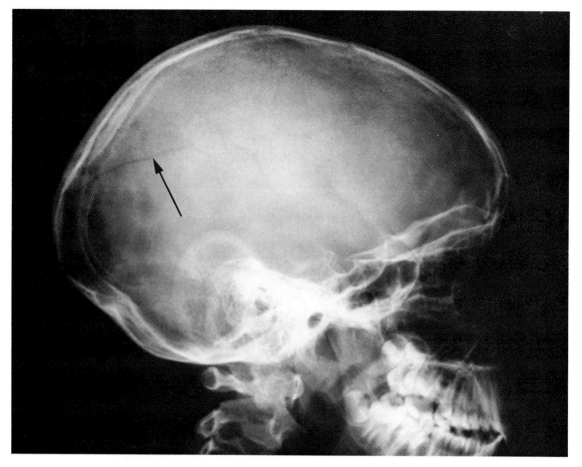

Fig. 6.24a   There is an extensive horizontal linear fracture (arrow) in the occipital bone through to the parietal bone in an older child.

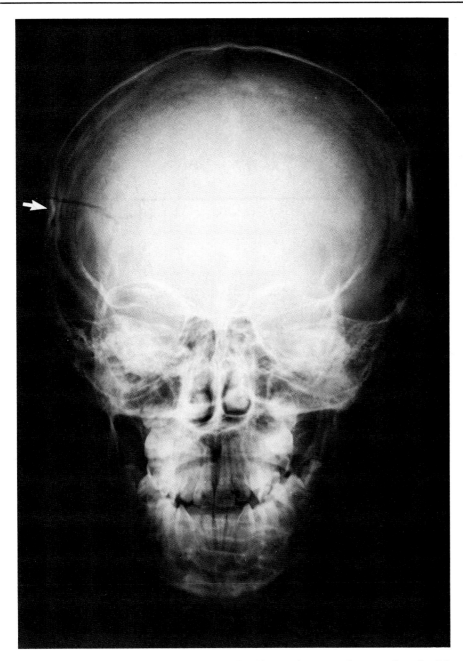

Fig. 6.24b   The frontal view shows the linear fracture is associated with mild bone depression adjacent to the linear fracture (arrow).

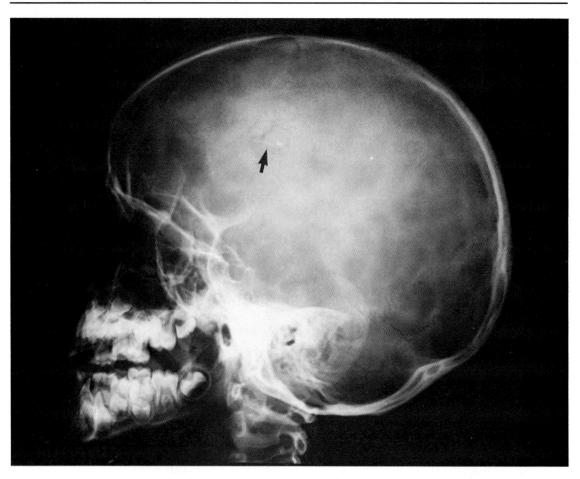

Fig. 6.25a   There is a small area indicating a depressed fracture (arrow) with radiating lines confined by a circular transradiant fracture line and minimal increased density.

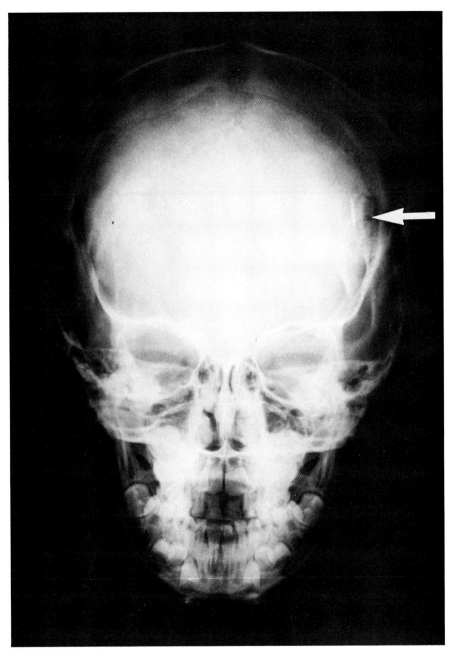

Fig. 6.25b The frontal view clearly shows the bone fragment (arrow) driven into the cranium of this child.

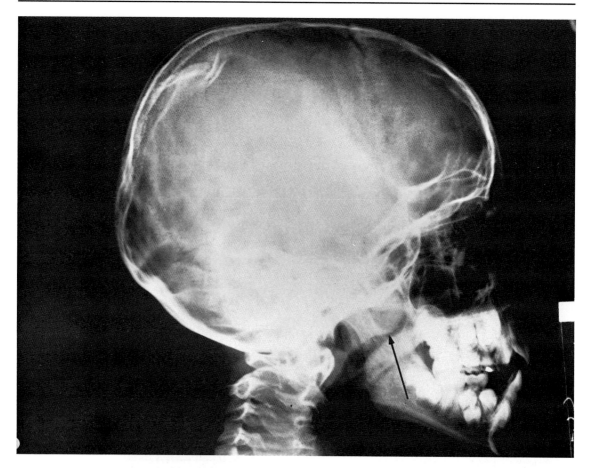

Fig. 6.26a Marked posterior parietal depressed fracture with bone fragments driven into the underlying cerebrum. There are marked prominent adenoidal soft tissues (arrow).

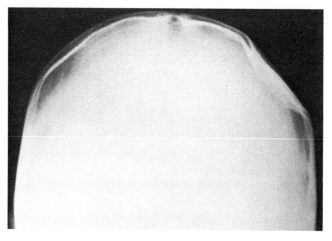

Fig. 6.26b The Towne's view shows the degree of flattening of the skull vault associated with the depressed fracture.

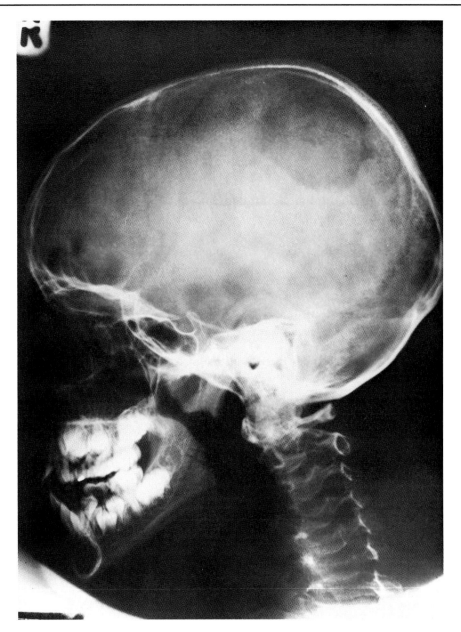

Fig. 6.26c   A film taken following surgery, showing the postsurgical defect at the site of the previous depressed fracture.

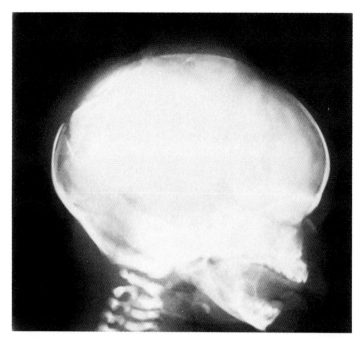

Fig. 6.27a   Gross macerated skull fracture of an infant tragically savaged by a dog. The infant subsequently died.

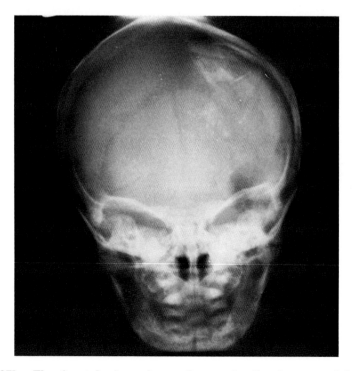

Fig. 6.27b   The frontal view shows the markedly depressed fracture indicating the degree of underlying brain damage.

Chapter 7

Fractures of the base of the skull

The demonstration of basal fractures with conventional radiography is extremely difficult and conventional tomography is invariably unhelpful. In the acute stage, basal views *must not be done* because the manipulation involved in examining the patient is hazardous, as the basal view demands full extension of the patient's neck: quite clearly a procedure contraindicated in an injured patient. Moreover the clinical signs are invariably definite enough to indicate the presence of a fracture, particularly blood or CSF from the ear, CSF rhinorrhoea or retroorbital haemorrhage, and, on routine views (Fig. 7.1), the presence of a fluid level in the sphenoidal sinus or a fracture line extending to the base of skull. In these circumstances, the patient must be immediately referred for a neurosurgical opinion and CT.

The demonstration of the base of the skull on CT shows fractures very clearly, whether through thick bone such as the petrous temporal or through the thin orbital plates (Figs. 7.2, 7.3). More importantly cerebral haemorrhage, oedema, space occupation with ventricular shift and intracranial gas are also clearly visible (Fig. 7.4). The use of basal views have thus largely been discontinued for patients attending accident and emergency departments.

It is therefore most important that the lateral projection should be made with a horizontal beam in order to reveal any air-fluid levels in sinuses or intracranially and to exclude air which may have entered the head as a result of a dural tear.

In spite of the limitations of conventional skull films, particularly in showing basal fractures, there are a number of radiographic signs to be noted:

(1) Air within the cranium
(2) Air-fluid level in air sinuses
(3) Fracture lines
(4) The basiocciput

AIR WITHIN THE CRANIUM

This indicates a dural tear and is best seen on the lateral, brow-up, horizontal beam projection (Fig. 7.5) as:

small bubbles over the frontal lobe
small bubble in the region of the chiasma
a large gas shadow over the cerebrum
an aerocele where there are dural adhesions, or
a spontaneous ventriculogram if there is a cerebral laceration

On the frontal view, a large gas shadow between the cerebral hemispheres may be shown.

AIR-FLUID LEVEL IN AIR SINUSES

If a fluid level is associated with trauma, it must be considered to indicate a basal fracture even though the fracture is not visible on skull radiographs. However, fluid levels in sinuses can also be due to incidental pathology such as sinusitis (see Figs. 8.10, 8.11).

FRACTURE LINES

Fractures of the base of skull (Fig. 7.6) are commonly accompanied by one or more fracture lines extending upwards into the bones of the vault from the petrous temporal or diagonally across the orbital plate and into the frontal bone. A fracture line extending to the base on conventional radiographs should be considered as a basal fracture until proved otherwise (Fig. 7.7).

Cranial nerve palsies may be secondary to compression by oedematous or displaced brain, such as third-nerve palsies caused by uncal herniation, or may be the result of a fracture involving a neural foramen, with local haematoma formation or direct nerve contusion. Computed tomography is required to show these fractures.

Non-infected intracranial gas collections are usually treated conservatively, but may be symptomatic and require more aggressive therapy, hence referral to a neurosurgical unit. Uncommonly, osteomyelitis may complicate a compound skull fracture while intracranial infection is an ever-present possibility with compound fractures that involve the subdural, epidural, or subarachnoid spaces. Meningitis or a brain abscess can result and, finally, localized gas accumulations may occur because of infection by gas-forming organisms.

Anterior fossa fractures are often an extension of a severe fracture of the frontal bone, involving the anterior walls of the frontal sinuses and continuing downwards across the orbital plate, also involving the roof of the ethmoids or posterior wall of the frontal sinus (Figs. 7.8, 7.9). Fractures in the squamous part of the frontal bone are seen more easily, but the cribriform plate fracture and the commonly associated CSF rhinorrhea complicating this fracture cannot be delineated, even though traditionally tomography in the coronal and lateral planes has been recommended for locating the exact site of the fracture. Computed tomography will invariably show the fractures of the thin orbital plate (Fig. 7.10) but fractures of the cribriform plate may not be shown. Conventional tomography is therefore no longer performed for CSF rhinorrhoea.

Sphenoidal fractures result from falls on the feet or vertex, and may extend across the lesser wings of the sphenoid or the walls of the optic canal. Blindness or lesser degrees of visual disturbance can result. Again CT is particularly useful with these fractures not usually visible on skull radiographs but indicated by the presence of an air-fluid level in the sphenoidal sinus (see Figs. 4.15, 6.21).

The oblique view of the optic formamina (Fig. 7.11) seldom shows the fracture whereas CT shows not only the fracture but soft-tissue changes within the orbit, such as haemorrhage, even in the absence of a fracture (Figs. 7.12–7.14). Deceleration accidents with sphenoidal fractures are also likely to be followed by CSF rhinorrhoea because the superior or lateral walls of the sphenoid sinus have been traumatized.

Following fractures of the sphenoid sinus there may be widening of the pre-sphenoidal nasopharyngeal soft tissues to greater than 16 mm in adults, shown on the lateral skull film. After fractures of the medial pterygoid plates the patient may be unable to close the mouth properly.

The petrous temporal bone

In severe head injuries, the ear is the most frequent sensory organ damaged, often resulting in hearing loss or facial paralysis. The petrous fracture is often not visible on plain films but detailed investigation of the middle ear is required because the disrupted ossicular chain can be reconstructed. Early referral of such patients to a specialist unit is mandatory where special views or high-definition CT for visualization of the fracture and the middle ear ossicles will be undertaken.

Fractures of the temporal bone that involve the bony labyrinth may be long-itudinal or horizontal. Longitudinal fractures run parallel to the long axis of the petrous bone but may also cross the tympanic cavity where the facial nerve may be injured. Conductive deafness can also occur as a result of ossicular displacement. As this can be treated surgically, it must be distinguished from transverse fractures of the bony labyrinth running laterally from the jugular fossa as such a fracture often results in complete and permanent sensorineural deafness. Testing for taste and lacrimation and of course facial movements must be done before any radiological investigation for traumatic facial palsy is undertaken, so that the examination may be concentrated on the segment of the nerve most likely to be damaged or compressed.

THE BASIOCCIPUT

The detection of intracranial haemorrhage in this region is clinically difficult and delays may lead to serious complications unless there is immediate operat-ive intervention. The detection of an occipital fracture is important as an indi-cation of early referral to a neurosurgical unit for CT (Fig. 7.15).

The occipital bone is best evaluated in the Towne's and lateral projections (Figs. 7.16, 7.17). The metopic suture of the frontal bone, as has been men-tioned earlier, can mimic a fracture but note the midline fracture of the occiput stops at the posterior lip of the foramen magnum on the Towne's view whereas the metopic suture will appear to 'extend' beyond the foramen magnum (Fig. 7.18).

The midline occipital fissure usually starts from the foramen magnum and should not extend more than 1–2 cm dorsally whereas the usual fracture in this area is linear and extends the length of the supraoccipital bone. Occipital fractures often have an oblique plane forming the 'beveled fracture' which shows as double lines (Figs. 7.19, 7.20). To complete the viewing of the base, fractures around the condyles must be remembered and basilar fractures extending into the pneumatized mastoid should be identified. Occasionally an unsuspected fracture of the upper cervical vertebrae may be diagnosed on the lateral and frontal skull projections (Fig. 7.21).

FURTHER READING

Tomsick T. A., Chambers A. A., Lukin R. R. (1978). Skull fractures. *Semin. Roent-genol.*, **13**, 27–36.

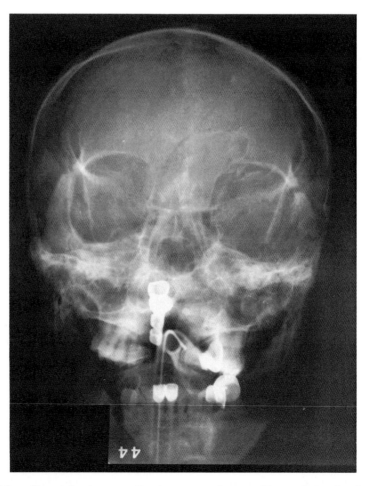

Fig. 7.1a Frontal view, patient unconscious with endotracheal tube. Long frontal fractures extend through the region of the frontal sinus. Diastasis of the left frontozygomatic suture and lateral orbital wall are also visible.

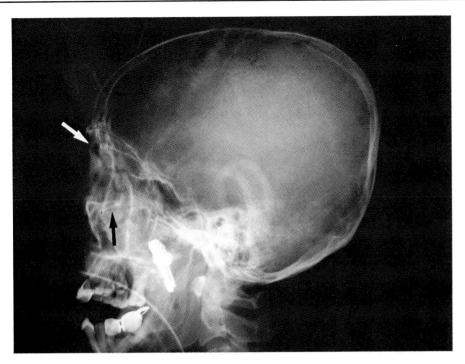

Fig. 7.1b The lateral view shows the fracture extending postero-inferiorly from the nasion towards the sphenoid sinus (white arrow) and also inferiorly to the orbital floor (black arrow).

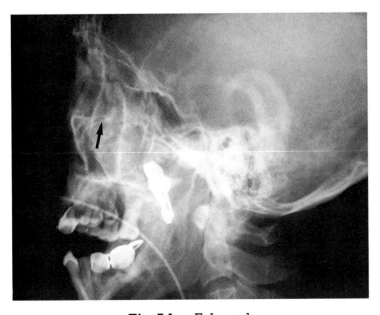

Fig. 7.1c Enlarged.

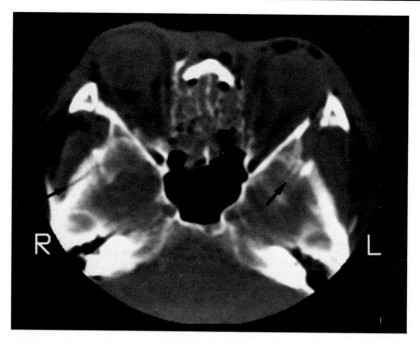

Fig. 7.2a   A CT section through the orbits showing gas in the soft tissues beneath the left eyelid, around the depressed nasal bone, in the right temporal fossa and small air-fluid levels in the ethmoidal sinuses. The fracture lines traverse the lateral orbital walls just posterior to the body of the zygoma and through the floor of the middle fossa (arrows).

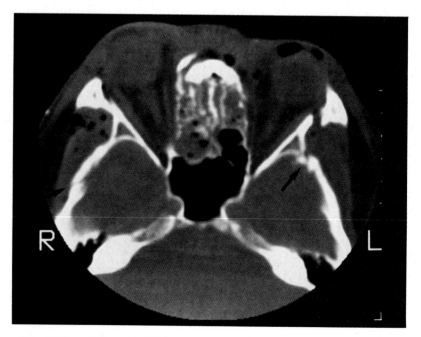

Fig. 7.2b   Adjacent CT section showing fracture lines (arrows).

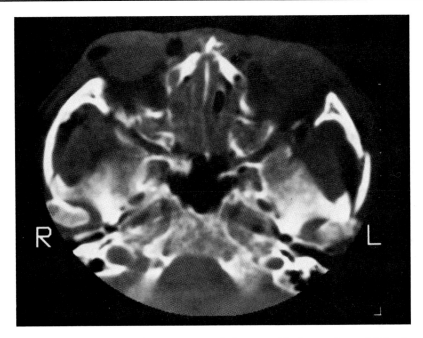

Fig. 7.3a   The fracture has separated the maxilla from the middle fossa just anterior to the pterygoid plate and has separated the zygomatic arches from the temporal bone.

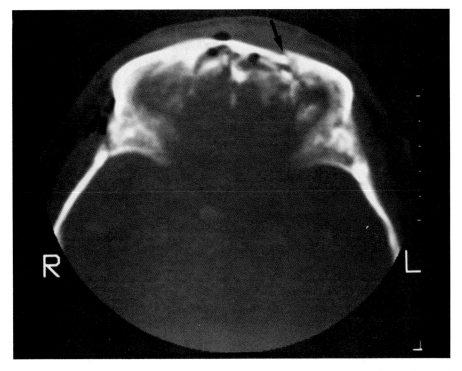

Fig. 7.3b   The frontal fracture passes through both walls of the frontal sinus (arrow).

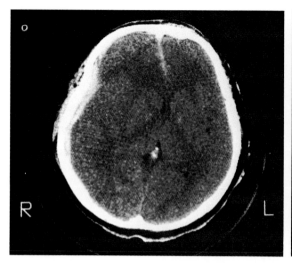 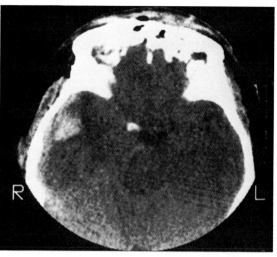

Fig. 7.4a There is moderate depression of the right parietal bone with a small acute subdural haematoma but also adjacent intracerebral haemorrhage with a markedly swollen right cerebral hemisphere and displacement of the midline structures towards the left.

Fig. 7.4b A CT section through a lower level. Note the right subdural haematoma is better shown here.

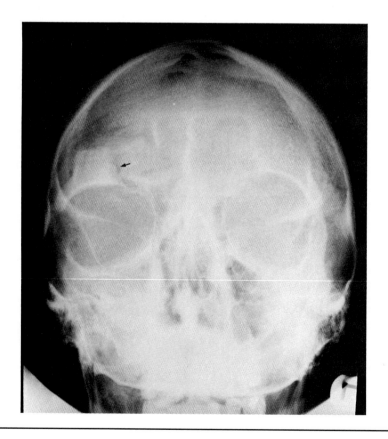

Below left:
Fig. 7.5a   A severe frontal fracture involving the superior orbital margin. The increased bone density of the fragments (arrow) indicates tilting of the bone and hence a depressed fracture. In addition the fracture involves the frontal sinuses.

Fig. 7.5b   The lateral view indicates that the posterior wall of the frontal sinus has been fractured (arrow) and there is gas within the cranium.

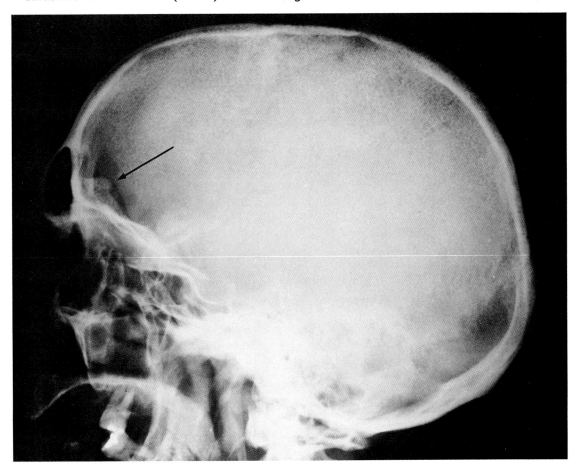

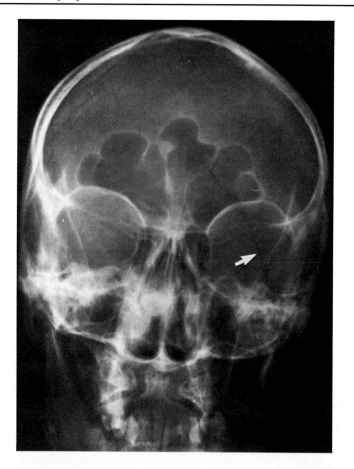

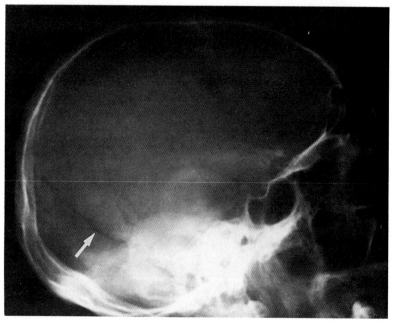

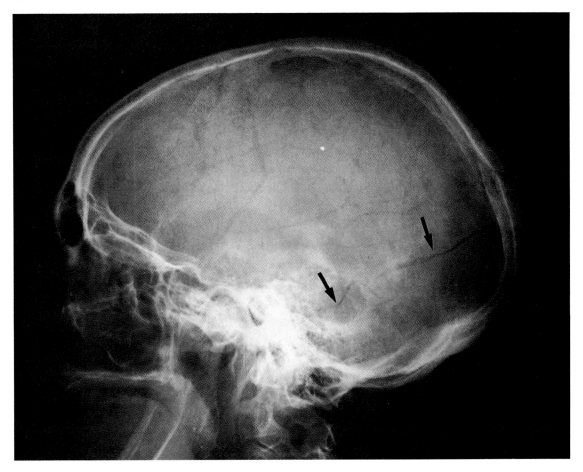

Fig. 7.7 A long, linear horizontal fracture of the left occipital bone extending to the skull base in the region of the mastoids (arrows). Further basal views or CT would be advised only if there was evidence of middle ear damage or neurological symptoms or signs. Haematomas of the posterior fossa are a dire emergency and must be decompressed immediately.

Top left:
Fig. 7.6a A posterior occipital fracture (arrow) extends downwards indicating basal involvement. It was not associated with symptoms, suggesting involvement of the petrous temporal.

Below left:
Fig. 7.6b The lateral view indicates that there is also suture diastasis (arrow).

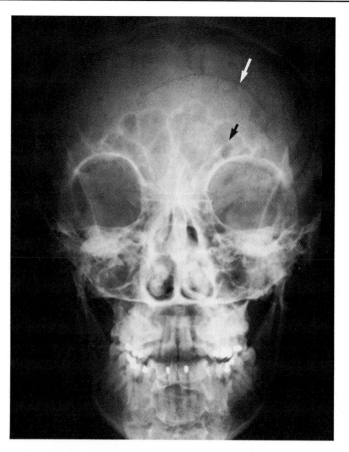

Fig. 7.8a   Obvious horizontal fracture (white arrow) but there is also a fracture of the frontal sinus with increased bone density of the fragment indicating depression (black arrow).

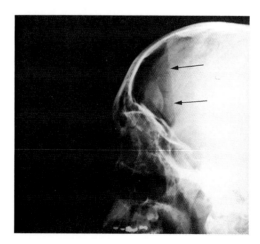

Fig. 7.8b   The fracture extends through the posterior wall of the frontal sinus with intracranial air and a large fluid level (arrows). The film was obviously taken with the patient supine and a horizontal x-ray beam.

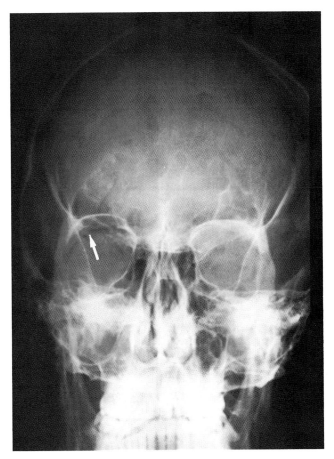

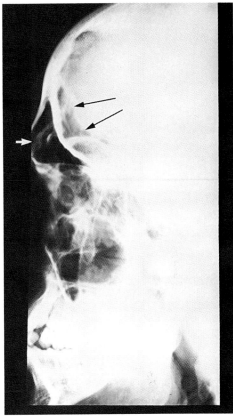

Fig. 7.9a Depressed fracture of the right superior orbital plate with gas in the orbit (arrow) indicating communication with the frontal sinuses.

Fig. 7.9b The fracture line in the frontal sinus (black arrows) is visible and there is intracranial gas. Loose bone fragments (white arrow) are visible within the frontal sinus.

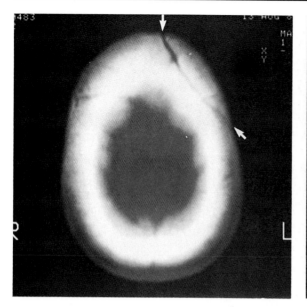

Fig. 7.10a   The linear fracture of the frontal bone can be seen extending to the vertex (arrow).

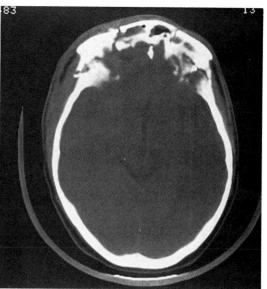

Fig. 7.10b   The frontal fractures extend to the superior orbital plates and the right fracture traverses the lateral margin of the right frontal sinus.

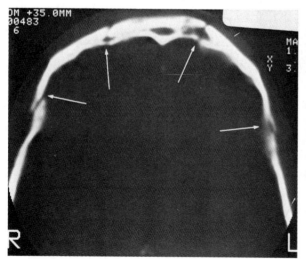

Fig. 7.10c   Axial CT shows multiple frontal bone fractures (arrows).

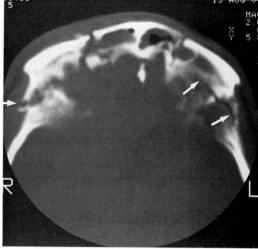

Fig. 7.10d   An enlarged view of the frontal region showing the fracture of the left superior orbital plate (long arrows) and the right lateral orbital wall (short arrow).

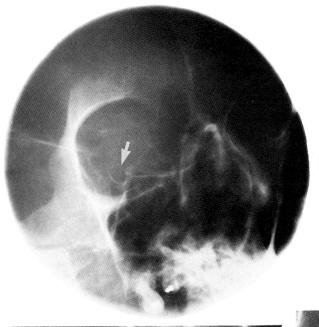

Fig. 7.11 Special view of the orbit to show the optic foramen (arrow).

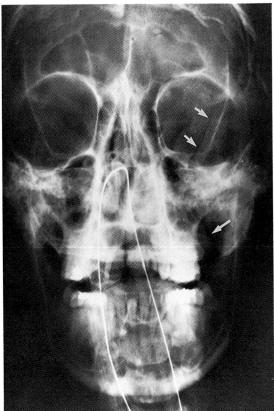

Fig. 7.12a Severe posterior fracture (arrows) in an unconscious patient.

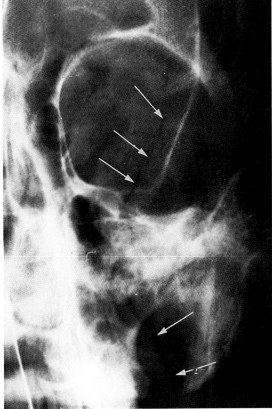

Fig. 7.12b The enlarged view shows the fracture (arrows), superimposed on the orbit, extending down to the skull base.

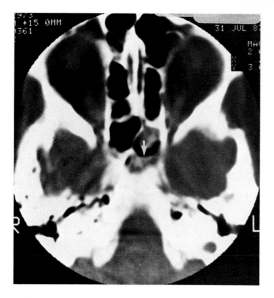

Fig. 7.12c Computed tomography of the base shows a fluid level in the sphenoidal sinus (arrow).

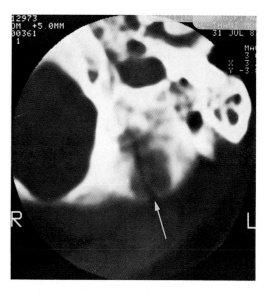

Fig. 7.12d There is also a clear indication of the fracture extending into the base adjacent to but not involving the foramen magnum (arrow).

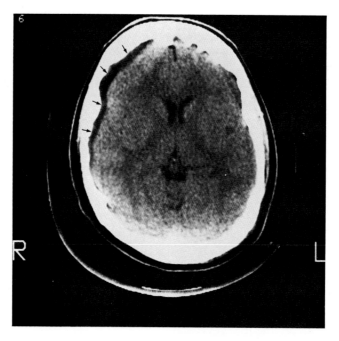

Fig. 7.12e A small right subdural haematoma (arrows) is clearly demonstrated but there is only slight associated space occupation.

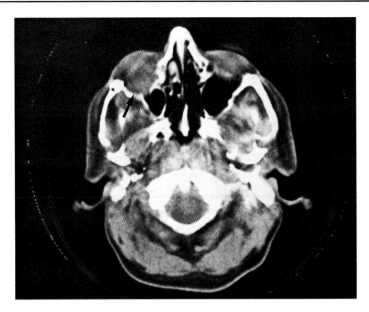

Fig. 7.13   A CT scan of a patient with post-traumatic proptosis. Note the retrobulbar haematoma (arrow).

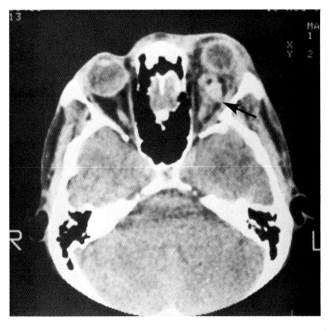

Fig. 7.14   A CT scan of a patient who has sustained a penetrating injury to the left eye. Note that the lens is not visible in the globe of the left eye and there is an extensive haematoma posterior to the globe (arrow).

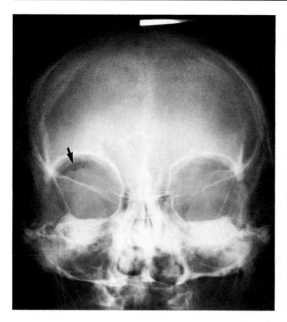

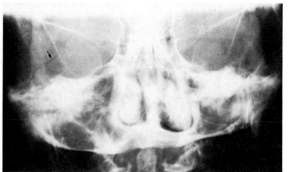

Fig. 7.15a   Gas is visible in the right orbit (arrow) following skull trauma.

Fig. 7.15b   A posterior occipital fracture has been shown projected through the right orbit (arrow).

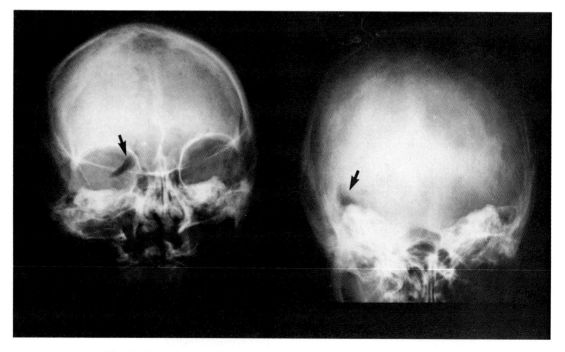

Fig. 7.15c   Gas is shown in the subtentorial region (arrows) on the frontal and Towne's views.

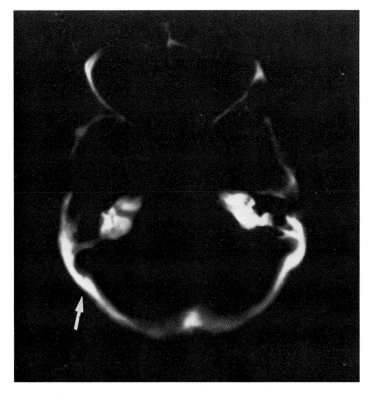

Fig. 7.15d   The CT scan shows the right occipital fracture.

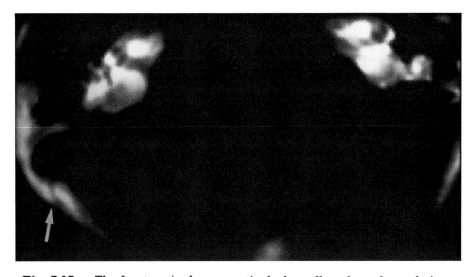

Fig. 7.15e   The fracture is shown particularly well on the enlarged view.

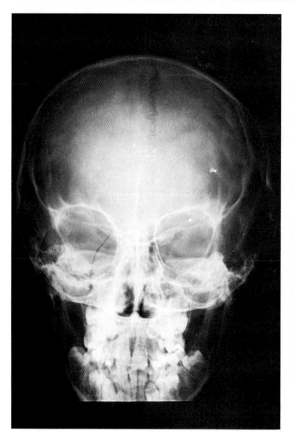

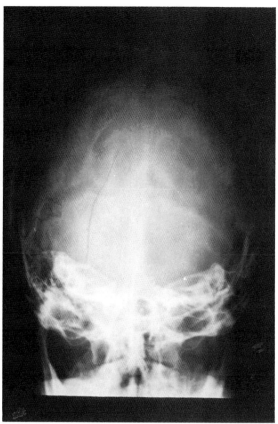

Fig. 7.16a There is a vertical fracture line superimposed on the right orbit, extending to the inferior margin of the posterior fossa, indicating an occipital fracture.

Fig. 7.16b The Towne's view clearly shows the vertical fracture extending to the skull base.

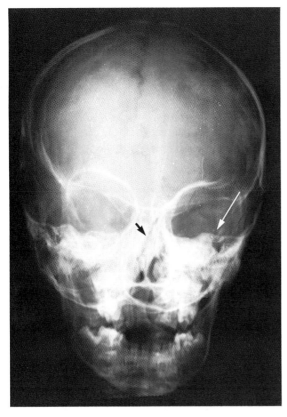 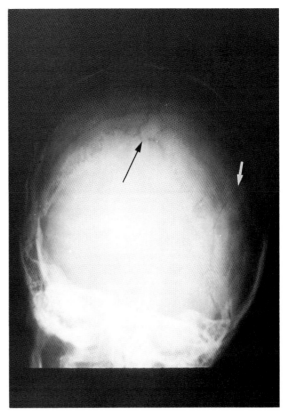

Fig. 7.17a Frontal view showing the occipital fractures superimposed on the left orbit and across the nose (arrows).

Fig. 7.17b Undertilted Towne's view showing a linear fracture of the left parietal bone extending into the lambdoid suture (white arrow). Wormian bones within the suture (black arrow) are also present.

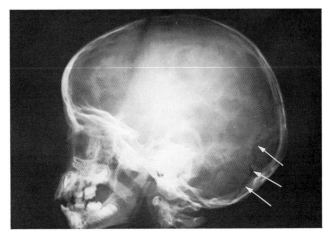

Fig. 7.17c Lateral view showing occipital fracture extending into the lambdoid suture (arrows).

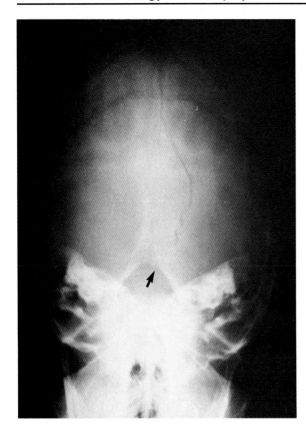

Fig. 7.18   The long vertical linear fracture of the occipital bone extends downwards to the left posterior margin of the foramen magnum (arrow).

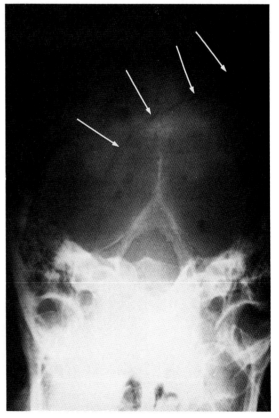

Fig. 7.19   A long occipital fracture (arrows) runs across the region of the internal occipital protuberance (torcula herophili). The multiple small lucencies are venous lakes.

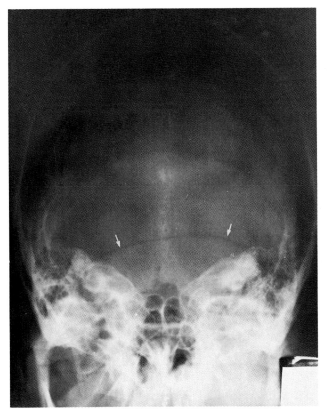 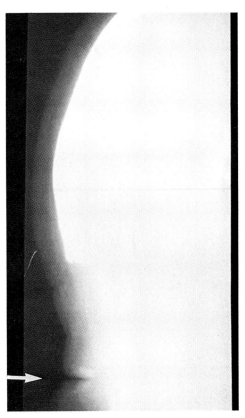

Fig. 7.20a A long transradiancy across the occipital bone (arrows) is not a fracture but due to gas trapped in a posterior skin fold associated with marked subcutaneous adiposity.

Fig. 7.20b The soft-tissue film on the lateral view demonstrates the skin fold well (arrow).

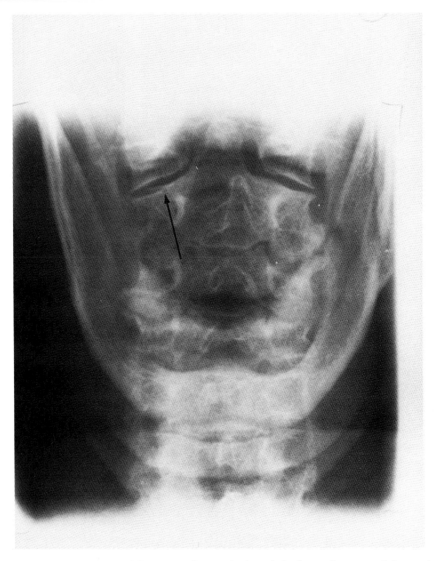

Fig. 7.21 Depressed fracture through the right lateral mass of the axis (arrow) in the frontal view of the cervical spine, first demonstrated on the skull film.

Chapter 8

Fractures of the facial bones

The facial skeleton can be divided into three areas: the upper third, formed by the frontal bone, the lower third, formed by the mandible, and the middle third, the area in between. Fractures in this region invariably result from direct injury, over 50% being caused by road traffic accidents, apart from isolated fractures of the nose.

RADIOGRAPHY

The routine 30° occipitomental (OM) view usually shows a fracture line if present but if there is any doubt, a 60° OM projection can be done (Fig. 8.1).

INTERPRETATION

The symmetry and alignment of the skull must be checked by following the contours along the following lines (McGrigor and Cambpell, 1950) (see Fig. 2.7b).

(1) From the zygomaticofrontal suture along the superior orbital ridges
(2) From the zygomatic arch along the inferior orbital margins
(3) From the inferior border of the zygomatic arch across the maxillary alveolus
(4) Along the superior border of the mandible
(5) Along the inferior border of the mandible, although this line will not be seen on a mouth-open OM projection

The OM view not infrequently shows the frontozygomatic synostosis very clearly, occasionally simulating fractures or diastasis (Fig. 8.2) but should not be confused with fractures as they are symmetrical, without any evidence of soft-tissue swelling, and isolated fractures are very uncommon.

The upper third

The common fractures in the upper third of the face are through the anterior wall of the frontal sinuses, usually a depressed fracture secondary to a direct blow (see Figs. 7.9, 7.10). As with other depressed fractures a tangential view is extremely useful and is easily achieved as a routine lateral projection but once again, must be supine, brow up with a horizontal x-ray beam so as not to miss an intracranial air-fluid level (see Fig. 7.8).

The middle third

The middle third of the face is further divided into a central region flanked by right and left lateral areas.

Fractures of the central region include those of the nasal bones not well demonstrated even by a local lateral, or the routine OM view but require the shooting-down view along the line of the nose onto an 'occlusal' film held between the lips by the patient (Figs. 8.3–8.6).

The lower third

Central fractures involving the maxilla (Le Fort) (Fig. 8.7) are due to much more severe injuries.

The Le Fort I is a transverse fracture of the maxilla across the apices of the teeth and base of nose. The fragment can often be felt to be free by moving it gently with a grip on the incisor teeth.

The Le Fort II fracture traverses the floors of the orbits through the maxillary antra starting at the nasal bones. An associated fracture of the cribriform plate with a tear of the dura mater often coexists with rhinorrhoea as a further complication (Figs. 8.8, 8.16).

The Le Fort III is a transverse fracture across the face, starting from one zygomatic arch and broadly sweeping to the other through the back of the orbits and the nose. The cribriform plate is usually fractured as well (Fig. 8.9).

Triple fractures of the malar bone occur from a direct blow to the cheek and are usually well demonstrated on OM and Towne's projections. On the OM view disruption of the frontozygomatic suture and clouding of the maxillary antrum are the predominant signs (Figs. 8.10, 8.11).

There are three degrees of injury. First is an uncomplicated fracture of the zygomatic arch or body without disturbance of mandibular movements (Figs. 8.12–8.14). Depression of the zygomatic arch, however, produces a bad cosmetic appearance, obviously requiring surgical intervention (Figs. 8.15–8.18). Secondly, disturbance of mandibular movement can occur as a complicating factor. Furthermore, an associated fracture of the lateral wall of the maxillary antrum may alter the position of the globe of the eyeball, causing double vision and hooding of the upper eyelid as it follows the globe downwards. Thirdly, there may also be a fracture of the orbital floor that can be confirmed and delineated by tomography or more adequately by CT, particularly in the coronal plane, showing the full extent of the soft-tissue injury (Figs. 8.19–8.24).

Fractures of zygomatic arches or mandibular condyles can occasionally be more adequately assessed with a submentovertical view but should not be requested in the acute stage; bearing that in mind, bony union occurs rapidly in facial bones, and therefore if left untreated for more than 21 days the deformity may well be uncorrectable.

BLOW-OUT FRACTURES OF THE ORBIT

These can have serious consequences; furthermore the recognition of the fracture can be quite difficult in many cases. A blow to the orbit by an object with a greater diameter than the orbital margins produces this fracture and forces the globe into the cone, resulting in some of the orbital contents being pushed through the floor. The fragment that hangs down from the floor thus gives rise to the 'teardrop' appearance (Figs. 8.25–8.31). In this process, the inferior rectus and inferior oblique muscles may be trapped, causing diplopia. Subsequently enophthalmos develops as the haemorrhage is absorbed, and as fibrosis takes the place of orbital fat. Surgery should be undertaken within 14 days if the previously mentioned complications are to be avoided.

The films taken soon after the injury may show orbital emphysema (Figs. 8.32–8.34) because of air, usually from a fracture of the walls of the ethmoidal air cells.

LATE COMPLICATIONS OF FACIAL FRACTURES

These include diplopia and obstructive epiphora. Fractures of the central middle third of the face involving the lacrimal fossa are particularly liable to damage the lacrimal sac and duct to produce the 'watery eye'.

The superior orbital fissure syndrome is a rare complication of fractures of the zygomatic complex caused by damage to the III, IV, and VI cranial nerves as they pass through the fissure; ophthalmoplegia, ptosis, proptosis, and a fixed dilated pupil results. The prognosis is poor although slow partial recovery may occur.

Mandibular movements will be limited if the coronoid process impinges on a depressed zygomatic bone, causing difficulty and pain on chewing and also late osteoarthrosis of the temporomandibular joint.

FRACTURES OF THE MANDIBLE

Radiographic views

(1) A PA projection of the mandible is the essential view but should be sup-
    plemented by one of the following projections
(2) A 30° oblique view of the body, angling the tube, for a view of each side
    in turn
(3) Orthopantomography (OPT) (Fig. 8.35) is a rotated PA projection of one
    or both sides but requires special apparatus
(4) Lateral tomography of the temporomandibular region
(5) Occlusal view of the anterior aspect of the body of the mandible

A fracture of the neck of the condyle is not infrequently overlooked as it tends to be hidden by overlying bone.

Radiography

The Towne's view usually shows the region of the mandibular condyle and neck of the mandible but lateral tomography may be required for an adequate demonstration of this area.

A blow on the symphysis menti may cause a fracture of the neck of the mandibular condyle, either unilateral or bilateral. The condyle is often displaced forwards and inwards by the external pterygoid muscle. The mouth is then held partially open with malocclusion on biting. If the diagnosis is delayed, there may be loss of some, if not all, of the teeth. In children, a fracture of the head and neck of the condyle will result in gross asymmetry of growth and ankylosis.

The ascending ramus usually fractures in the region of the angle of the jaw on the side of the blow and is usually associated with a fracture of the neck of the opposite condyle or a fracture of the opposite horizontal ramus in the region of the root of the canine tooth.

The body of the jaw bone is the most common fracture of the mandible and is usually a bilateral or double fracture occurring at the canine tooth sockets (Fig. 8.36). The teeth in the line of fracture should be identified since they are a potential source of infection.

Orthopantomography gives a complete view of the mandible and teeth (Fig. 8.35) but requires special apparatus not always available. Cooperation of the patient is also required and therefore has limited application in the immediate management of head injuries.

The temporomandibular joints (TMJ) will only be mentioned briefly because the diagnosis and management of the TMJ are primarily the responsibility of the oral surgeons and the mainstay of diagnosis is a detailed and specialized radiological examination.

The common abnormality seen in accident and emergency departments is a bilateral dislocation usually occurring after a rather vigorous, uncontrolled yawn (Fig. 8.37). The mandibular condyles ride high in front of the temporal articular eminence, with the intraarticular disc behind being locked out, preventing a normal return. Radiography is usually unnecessary unless a superadded fracture is suspected.

REFERENCE AND FURTHER READING

McGrigor D. B., Cambpell W. (1950). The radiology of war injuries. *Br. J. Radiol.*, **23**, 685.

Rowe N. L., Killey H. C. (1968). Fractures of the facial skeleton, 2nd edn. Edinburgh: Churchill Livingstone.

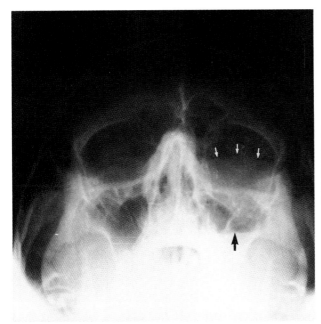

Fig. 8.1a 'Teardrop' blow-out fracture of the left inferior orbital margin with a fluid level in the left maxillary antrum (black arrow) and soft-tissue swelling over the inferior aspect of the orbit (white arrows).

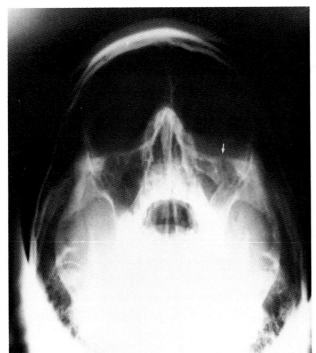

Fig. 8.1b An OM view with more tilt, i.e. the chin is higher, emphasizing the bone margins, the marked depression of the left orbital floor and the fracture (arrow), but the fluid level in the left maxillary antrum has disappeared, no longer being tangential to the x-ray beam.

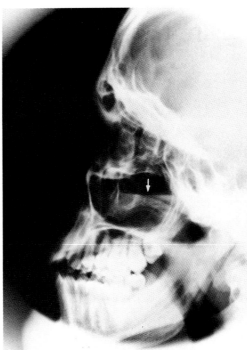

Fig. 8.1c On the lateral view, the fluid level is well demonstrated (arrow).

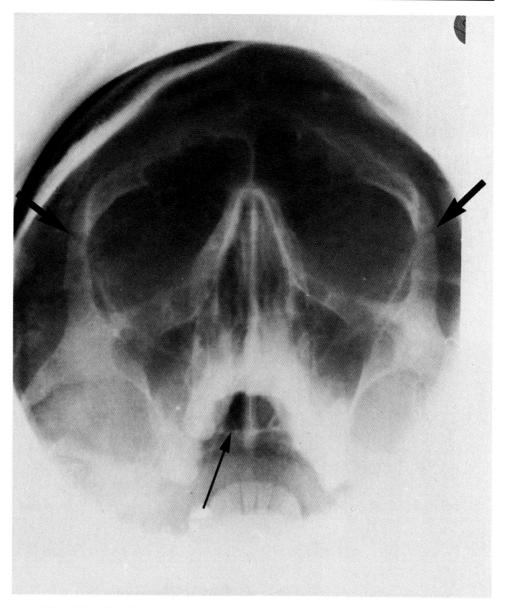

Fig. 8.2   An OM view with open mouth shows the sphenoid sinus (long arrow). Prominent zygomaticofrontal synostoses are also present (bold arrows), bilateral and symmetrical, not to be mistaken for fractures.

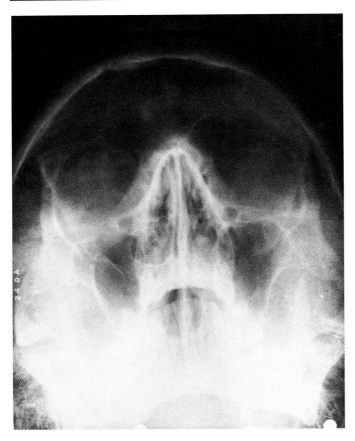

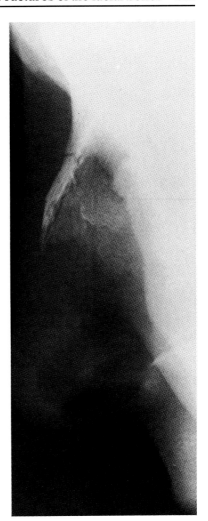

Fig. 8.3a   An OM view for nasal trauma. No fracture is visible and the antra are normally transradiant.

Fig. 8.3b   Lateral view of the nose with transradiant lines possibly representing fractures.

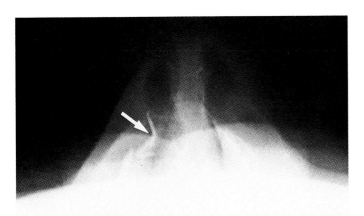

Fig. 8.3c   The shooting-down view clearly shows the fracture and buckling of the right nasal bone (arrow) requiring surgical realignment.

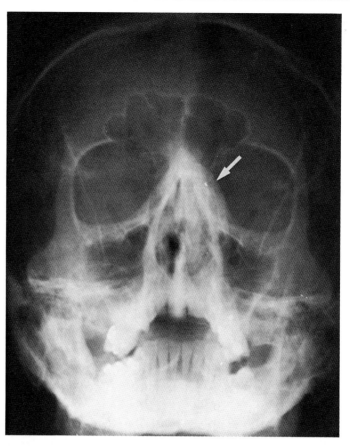

Fig. 8.4a Frontal view showing gross soft-tissue swelling to the left of the nose (arrow) and the left nasal cavity is opaque. However, no fracture is demonstrated on this view.

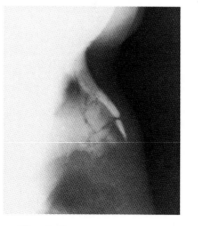 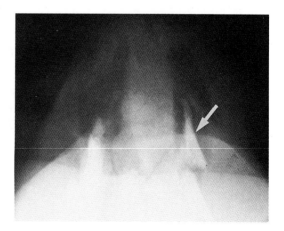

Fig. 8.4b Lateral view showing a comminuted nasal fracture with lateral displacement of the left nasal bone.

Fig. 8.4c Shooting-down view showing the fracture (arrow).

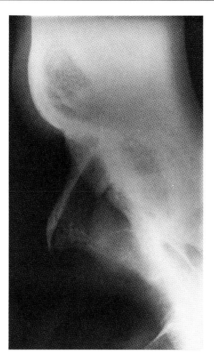

Fig. 8.5a   Lateral view of nose: no definite fracture is visible.

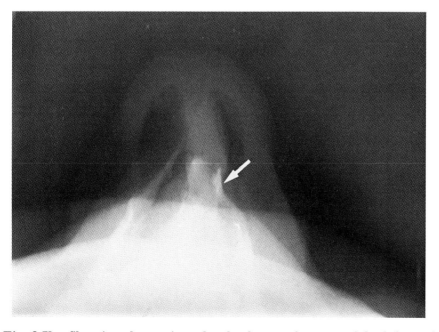

Fig. 8.5b   Shooting-down view clearly shows a fracture of the left nasal bone with marked depression (arrow) likely to produce a bad cosmetic result unless corrected.

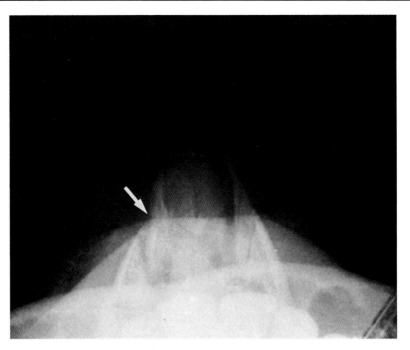

Fig. 8.6a   Shooting-down view of the nose showing a linear fracture of the right nasal bone with quite marked medial depression (arrow). A bad cosmetic appearance will result unless the bone is realigned.

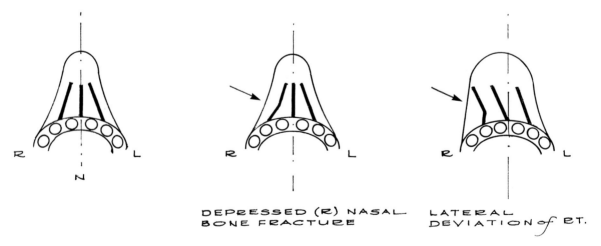

DEPRESSED (R) NASAL
BONE FRACTURE   LATERAL
                      DEVIATION of RT.

Fig. 8.6b   Diagram of shooting-down view of the nose.

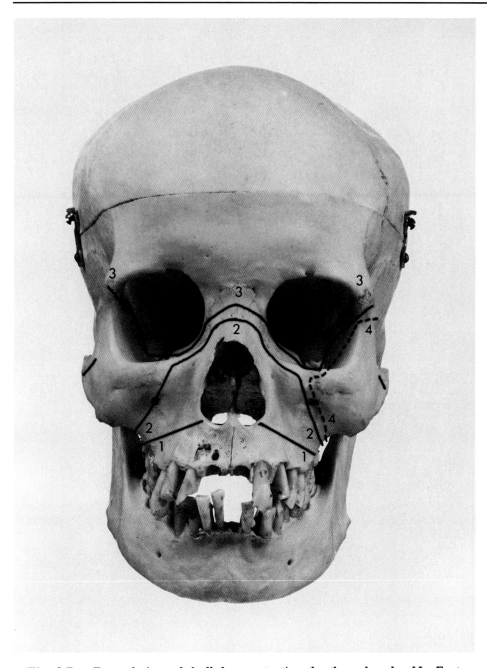

Fig. 8.7a   Frontal view of skull demonstrating the three levels of Le Fort fractures.

1. Le Fort I fracture
2. Le Fort II fracture
3. Le Fort III fracture
4. Line of triple fractures of the zygoma
(Note: the larger the number in Le Fort fractures, the 'higher' the fracture.)

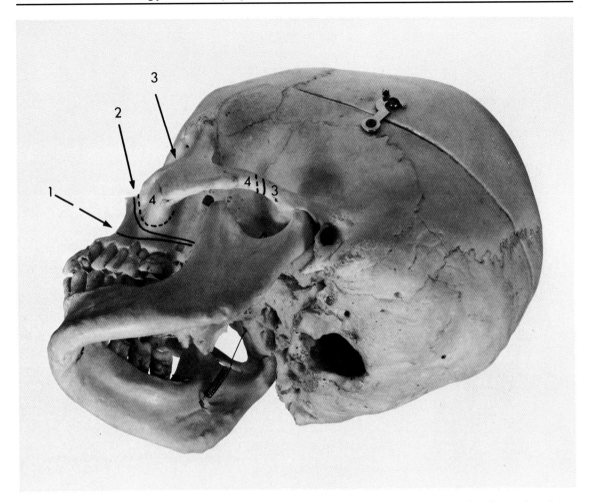

Fig. 8.7b   Oblique lateral view of skull demonstrating the three levels of Le Fort fractures and line of fractures of the zygoma (for key see Fig. 8.7a).

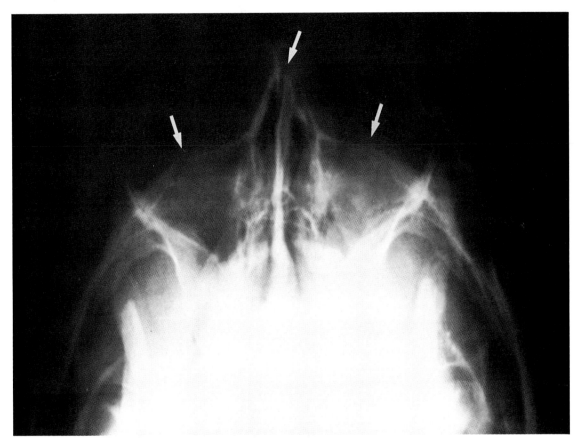

Fig. 8.8 An undertilted basal view to show the fractures (arrows) through the inferior orbital margins and nose in a Le Fort II facial fracture.

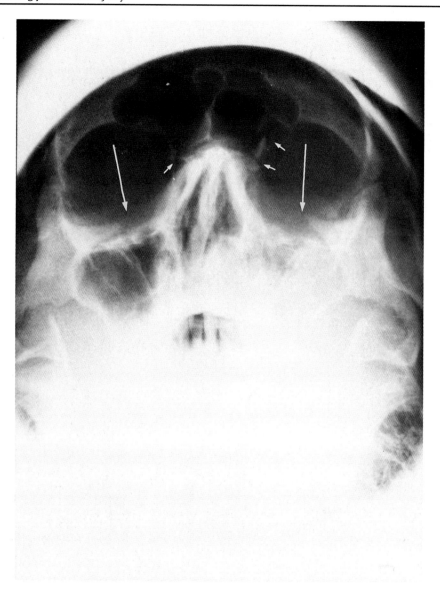

Fig. 8.9a A severe facial fracture (Le Fort III) through the bridge of the nose (small arrows) and orbital margins (long arrows) with an opaque left antrum. There is marked depression of the left inferior orbital margin.

Top right:
Fig. 8.9b On this less tilted OM view, the fracture (arrows) across the bridge of the nose is better demonstrated than in the previous view, though the fractures around both the inferior orbital margins are not clearly seen.

Below right:
Fig. 8.9c The lateral view demonstrates the fluid level (arrow) in the maxillary antrum very well.

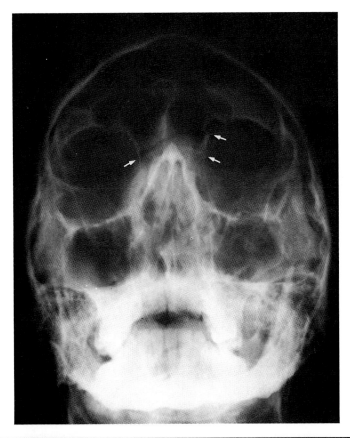

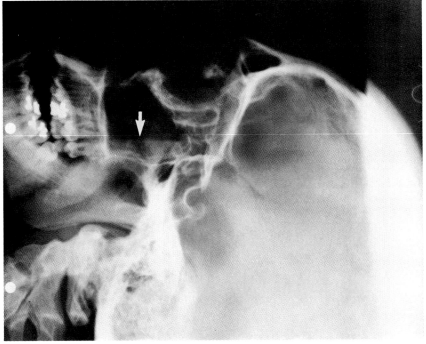

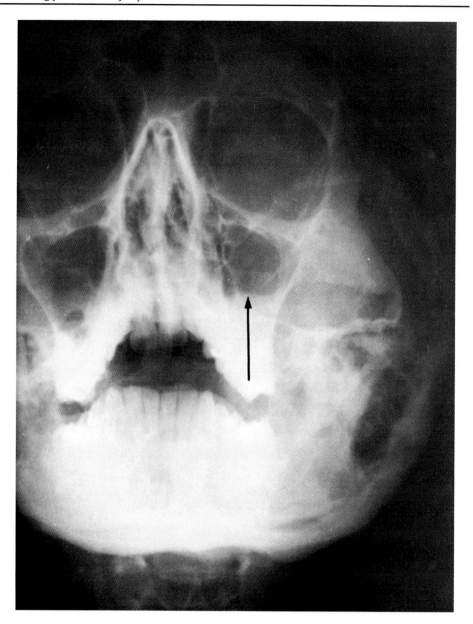

Fig. 8.10   The left antrum shows a fluid level (arrow) after trauma, but no fracture is visible. A fracture should be assumed although antral fluid can be caused by sinusitis.

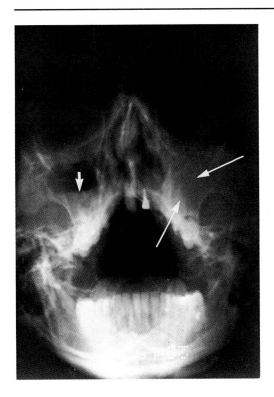

Fig. 8.11a The left antrum (long arrows) is opaque and there is a large fluid level in the right antrum (short arrow), probably due to sinusitis as the trauma was slight and away from the face.

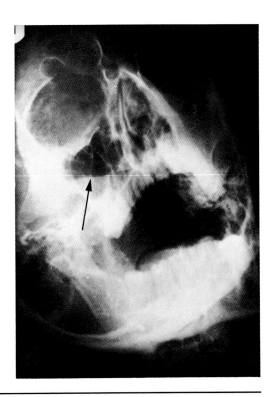

Fig. 8.11b The tilted view, no longer considered necessary, clearly shows the right antral fluid level (arrow).

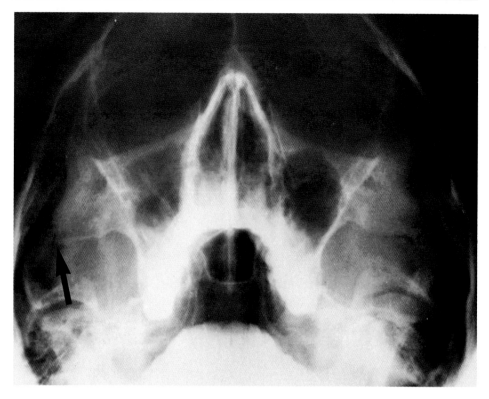

Fig. 8.12   An OM view showing undisplaced fracture of the right zygoma (arrow).

Top right:
Fig. 8.13a   A fracture of the lateral wall of the maxilla (short arrow) is associated with a linear fracture of the zygomatic arch (long arrow). The right antrum is opaque compared to the left.

Below right:
Fig. 8.13b   Close-up view showing the fractures of the zygoma (arrow).

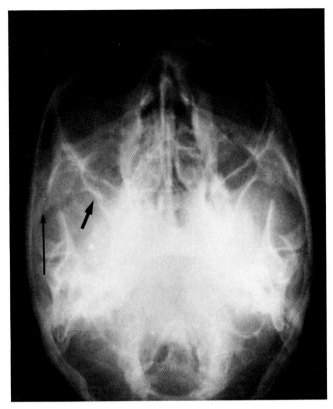

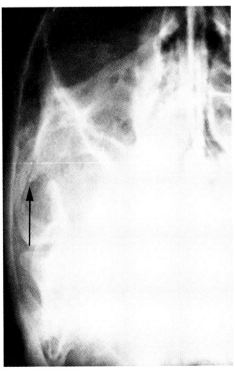

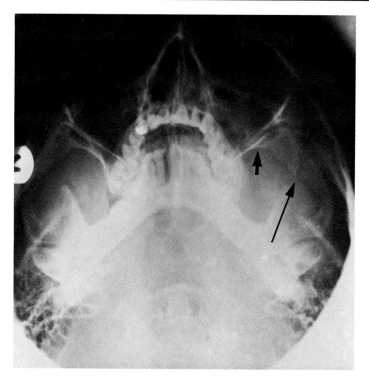

Fig. 8.14 Undisplaced fracture of the left zygoma (long arrow) and lateral wall of the antrum (short arrow). The fracture line extends into the body of the zygoma.

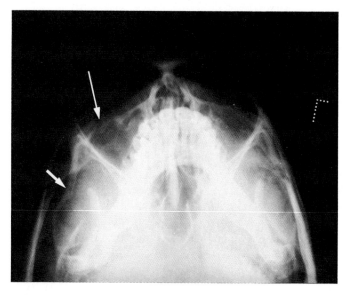

Fig. 8.15 There is marked depression (short arrow) of the right zygomatic arch due to a buckled fracture and a fracture of the inferior orbital margin (long arrow) indicating four distinct fractures. Unless corrected, a bad cosmetic effect will result.

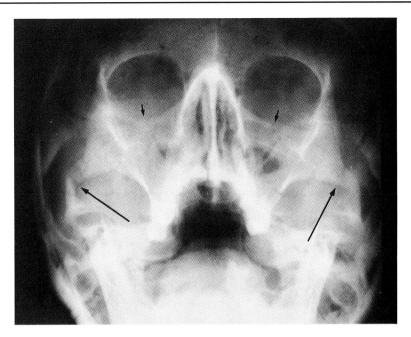

Fig. 8.16 Le Fort II fracture with opaque right antrum and a fluid level in the left antrum. Fractures of the inferior orbital margins (small arrow). Fractures of the zygomatic arches (long arrows).

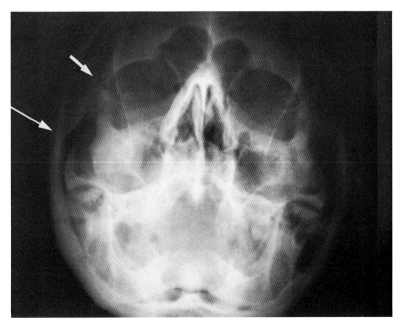

Fig. 8.17 Depressed fracture of the right zygoma (long arrow) with suture diastasis at the frontozygomatic arch (short arrow). The right antrum is opaque.

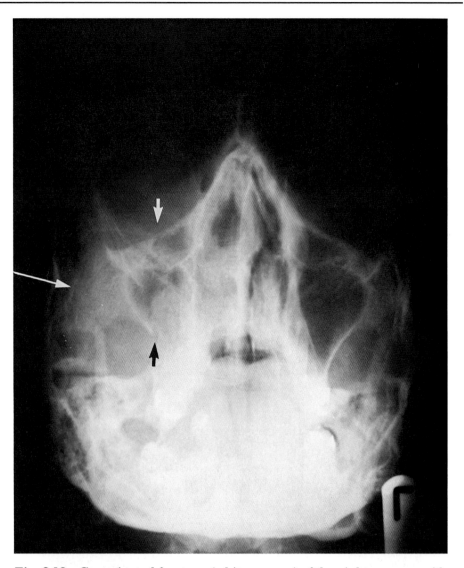

Fig. 8.18   Comminuted fracture (white arrows) of the right zygoma with the medial component running vertically through the antrum. In the right nasal cavity the ethmoidal sinuses and antrum are markedly opaque, indicating the extent of the soft-tissue injury. The body of the zygoma is displaced inwards (black arrow).

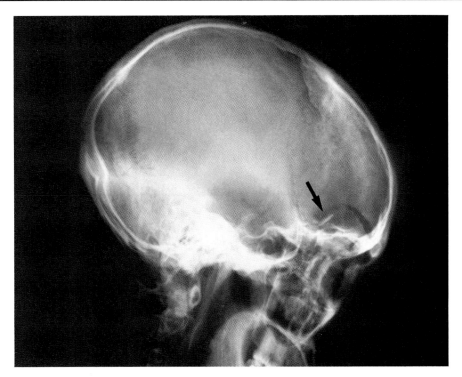

Fig. 8.19a The lateral view of a depressed fracture of the zygoma and superior orbital margin with a separated posterior bone fragment (arrow) and wide gap anteriorly.

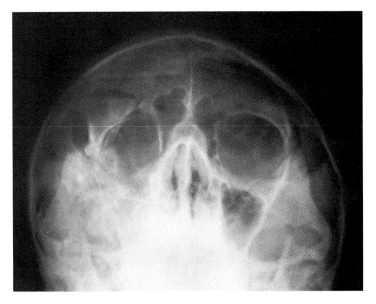

Fig. 8.19b The OM view shows the shattered zygoma and depressed superior orbital margin.

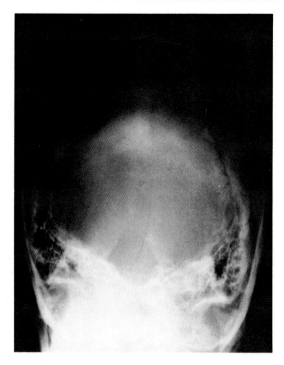

Fig. 8.20   The long vertical fracture must be through the frontal bone as it crosses the posterior margin of the foramen magnum overlying the foramen itself.

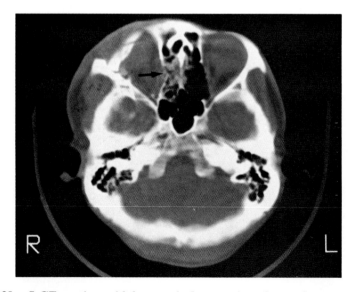

Fig. 8.21   A CT section with bone window setting shows the comminuted depressed fracture of the superior orbital margin, also a fracture through the posterior wall of the orbit and lateral wall of the ethmoids with partial opacification of the sinuses (arrow).

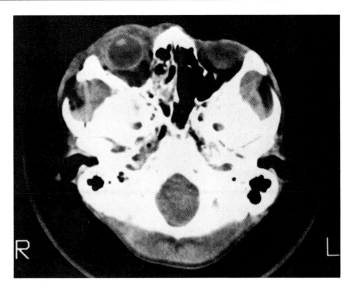

Fig. 8.22   There is a large haematoma around the anterior aspect of the right globe and partial opacification of the right ethmoidal sinuses.

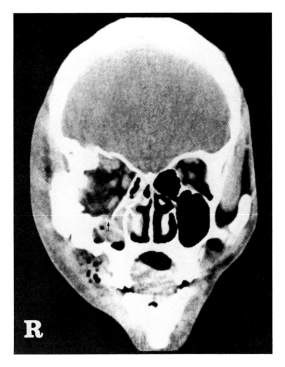

Fig. 8.23   Coronal CT section with soft-tissue setting showing the large right subcutaneous haematoma extending from the temporal bone down to the chin. The maxillary antrum is partially opacified due to a haematoma. A fracture of the inferior orbital margin is also visible (arrow).

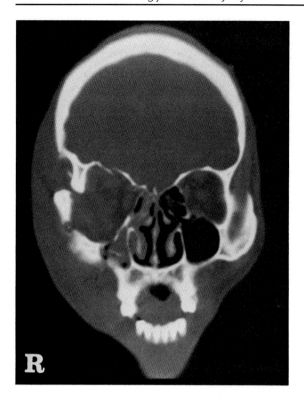

Fig. 8.24a Bone window setting of a CT coronal section 1 cm posteriorly shows the laterally displaced bone fragment separated from the frontal bone superiorly and body of the zygoma inferiorly. The fractures of the superior orbital margin are also visible. The right antrum is opaque with a large subcutaneous haematoma of the right side of the face.

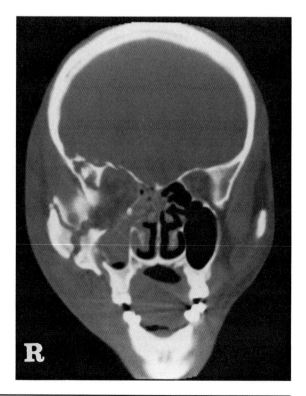

Fig. 8.24b A section further posteriorly shows the comminuted fracture of the body of the zygoma with multiple separated fragments and a comminuted fracture of the lateral margin of the superior orbital ridge. The ethmoidal sinuses and right antrum are opaque.

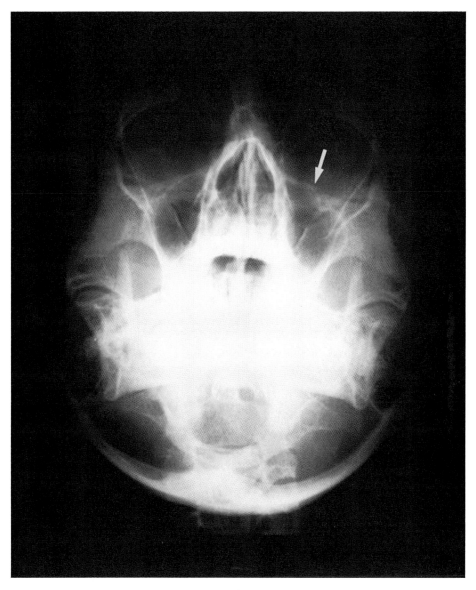

Fig. 8.25   There is a fracture of the left inferior orbital margin with down-ward tilt of the bone indicating a 'blow-out' fracture.

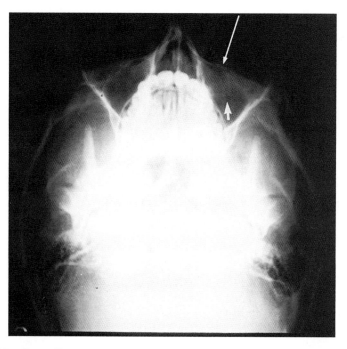

Fig. 8.26   Overtilted orbital view with a fracture of the inferior orbital margin (long arrow) and tilting of the bone indicating a blow-out fracture (short arrow).

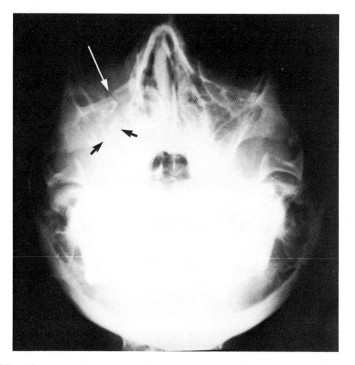

Fig. 8.27   Blow-out fracture of the inferior orbital margin (white arrow) with an opaque right antrum (black arrows).

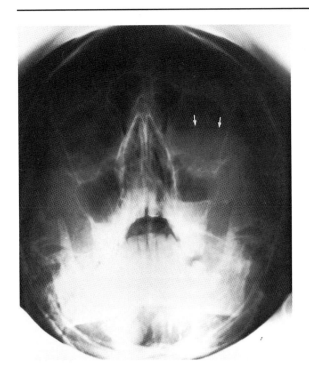

Fig. 8.28a There is a blow-out fracture of the left inferior orbital margin with an obvious fluid level in the left antrum. Inferior orbital soft-tissue swelling is also present (arrows).

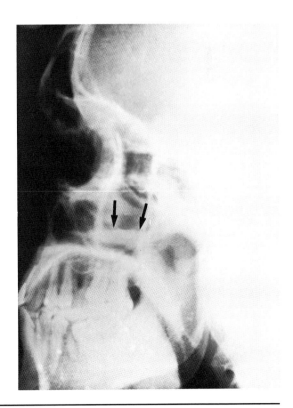

Fig. 8.28b A fluid level is present in the left antrum (arrows) following trauma, but the fracture of the inferior orbital margin was not visible on this view.

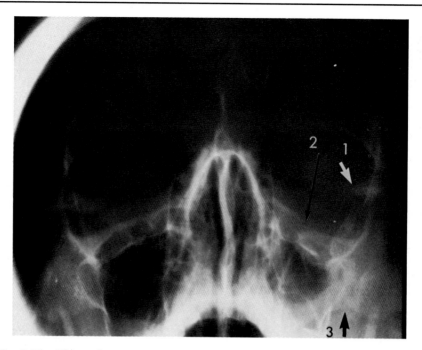

Fig. 8.29   There is a comminuted fracture of the left zygoma involving the body (3) and extending upwards into the frontal process (1) with a fracture through the inferior orbital margin and fluid in the inferior aspect of the left antrum. The inferior orbital margin is markedly tilted, indicating a blow-out fracture (2).

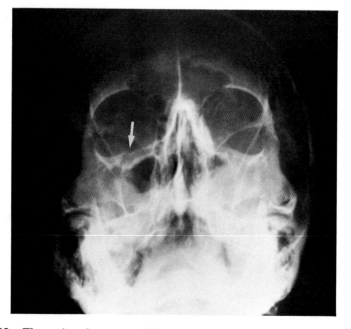

Fig. 8.30   There is a fracture of the right inferior orbital margin (arrow) with mucosal swelling and a fluid level in the right antrum. The left antrum is also opaque.

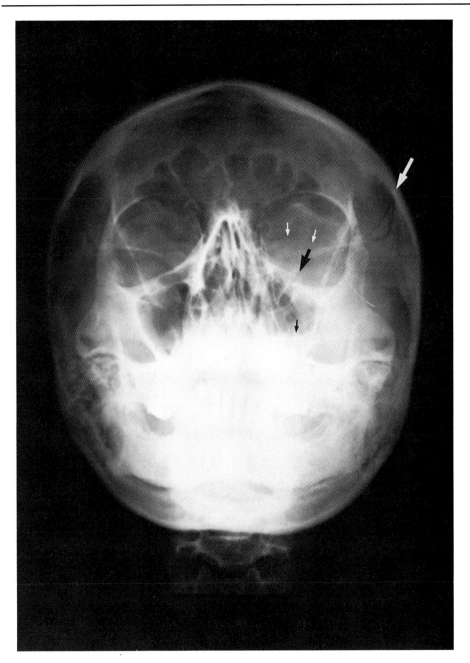

Fig. 8.31 Fracture of the left temporal bone (large white arrow), soft-tissue swelling in the orbit (small white arrows) and a fracture of the inferior orbital margin (large black arrow) with a fluid level in the left antrum (small black arrow).

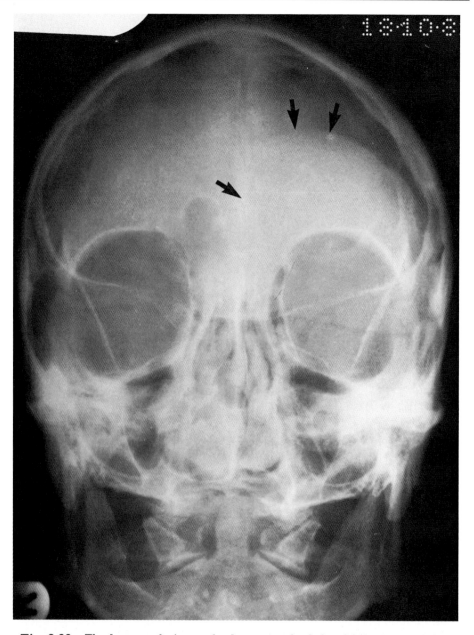

Fig. 8.32 The large soft-tissue shadow over the left orbit (arrows) is due to a haematoma following trauma, but it did not cause a fracture.

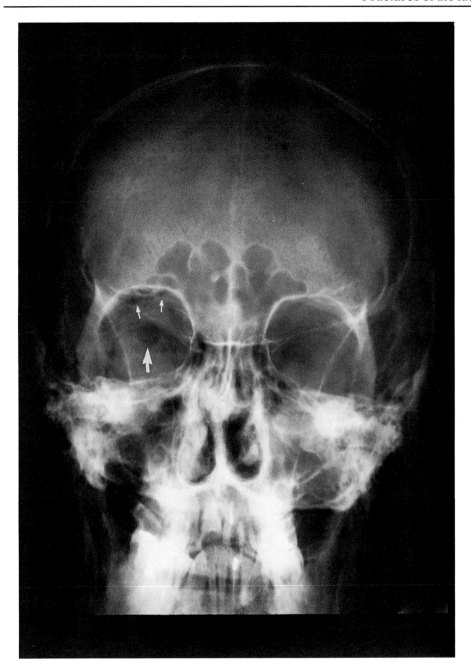

Fig. 8.33   Surgical emphysema of the right orbit (small arrows) with air trapped within the muscular conus (large arrow).

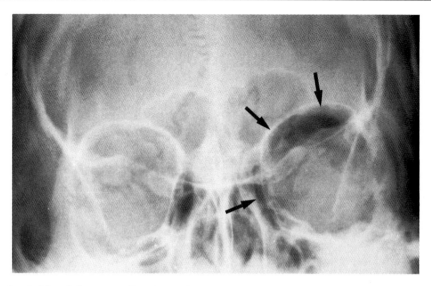

Fig. 8.34 A large collection of gas is present in the left orbit (arrows) on the superior and medial aspects indicating a fracture of the ethmoidal walls (arrow).

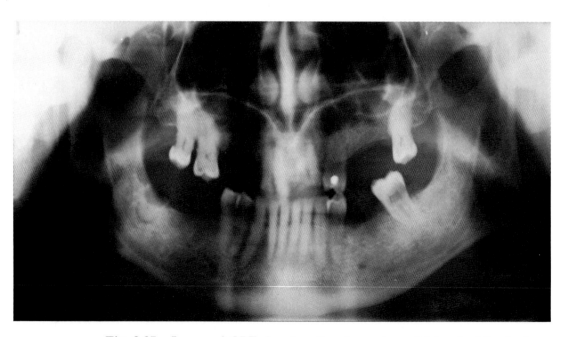

Fig. 8.35 A normal OPT showing the clear view obtained of the body of the mandible and lower incisor roots.

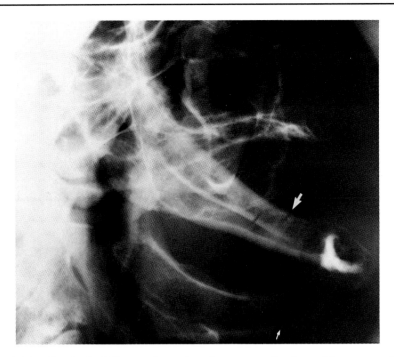

Fig. 8.36 Angled oblique view showing an undisplaced fracture of the horizontal ramus (large arrow). There is also a fracture of the opposite ramus in a similar position (small arrow).

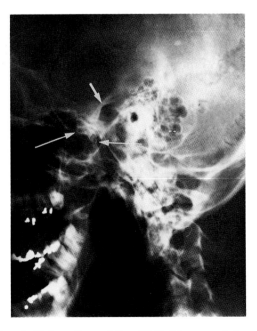

Fig. 8.37 Bilateral dislocation of the TMJ. The condyle of the mandible (long arrows) lies anterior to the articular eminence, with a bare articular fossa (short arrow) posteriorly just in front of the external auditory meatus. The mouth is wide open and fixed in this position.

Chapter 9

Normal variants, postsurgical appearances and foreign bodies

The importance of artefacts and normal variants lies in the diagnostic confusion caused particularly in recognizing fractures and in diagnosing pathology where none is present.

NORMAL VARIANTS

A prominent but normal diploic pattern of the calvarium (Fig. 9.1) is quite common and must not be mistaken for the 'pepper-pot' appearance of diffuse bone loss as occurs with hyperparathyroidism or other osteopenic conditions (Fig. 9.2).

Prominent 'digital' or 'thumbprint' impressions on the calvarium producing a 'copper-beaten' appearance are extremely variable and a quite common but normal finding in children, especially between four and ten years of age (Figs. 9.3, 9.4). Raised intracranial pressure should not be diagnosed simply on the basis of this observation (Fig. 9.5).

Burr holes (Figs. 9.6–9.8), surgical defects (Figs. 9.9, 9.10), Paget's disease (Figs. 9.11–9.14) and congenital parietal defects are readily recognized and must be distinguished from calvarial metastases (Figs. 9.15–9.17). An adequate history is paramount but the radiographic appearances are reasonably characteristic. Posterior or occipital venous lakes (Fig. 9.18 and see Fig. 3.8) fall into the same category and should not be mistaken for 'lytic bone' lesions as they are bilateral and near the midline on both sides, with irregular but well defined margins, and are most common in the elderly.

Bridging of the sella due to calcification of the interclinoid ligaments (Figs. 9.19 and 9.20) is not uncommon and does not relate to sellar diseases or other pathological conditions (Fig. 9.21). However, a large pituitary fossa (Fig. 9.22) must not be overlooked as a pituitary tumour may well cause blindness, mental clouding or even loss of consciousness and among other conditions can be associated with myxoedema due to hypothyroidism and acromegaly.

Hyperostosis frontalis is a common normal finding in the elderly in which there is extra ossification in both frontal bones; it has been discussed previously (see Chapter 3).

ARTEFACTS AND FOREIGN BODIES

Many artefacts in the hair and soft tissues of the head may be responsible

for linear lucencies, occurring quite commonly in neonates because of air trapped in skin folds, particularly in the scalp and nape of the neck, and also in
obese adults (see Fig. 7.20).

Artefacts commonly producing opaque shadows include foreign bodies
(Figs. 9.23–9.25), dirt, hair, and coagulated blood. Important above all are
fragments of glass lodged in the skin as a source of infection and non-healing
of a laceration. Glass from the windscreen of a motor vehicle is the commonest
source (Figs. 9.26–9.32), other foreign bodies such as surgical clips after
neurosurgery (Figs. 9.33, 9.34) and shunts used in decompression of hydro-
cephalus (Fig. 9.35), are more easily recognized. Occasionally, however, a
foreign body can produce a most unusual appearance such as the inner tube
of a ball-point pen seen end on (Fig. 9.36).

After careful examination of the scalp and removal of all possible opacities
from hair and clothing, further films are taken in an attempt to resolve any
difficulties. Further projections to localize the foreign body can then be
requested provided there has been adequate consultation to exclude
pathognomonic appearances such as blood in the hair (Figs. 9.37–9.40),
osteomas (see Fig. 3.15) and normal variants (Figs. 9.41–9.45).

FURTHER READING

Keats T. E. (1973). *An Atlas of Normal Roentgen Variants That May Simulate Disease*,
    pp. 5–65. Chicago: Year Book.

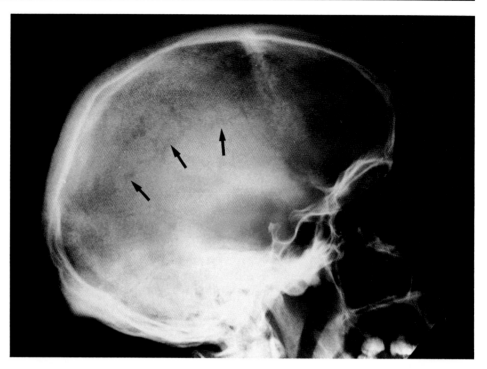

Fig. 9.1 Normal skull with 'pepper-pot' appearance of the superior cranium and prominent venous markings (arrows).

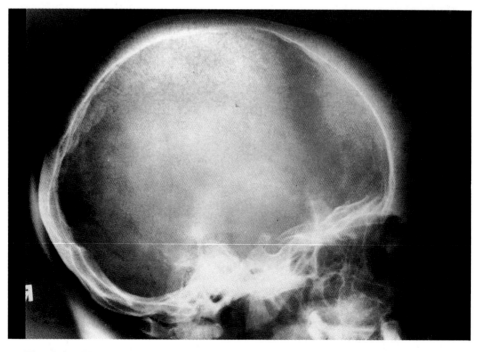

Fig. 9.2 Thickened cranium in a patient with haemopoietic (sickle cell) disease.

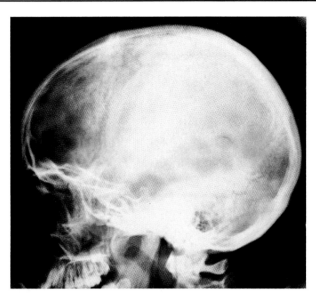

Fig. 9.3   The thumbprint lucencies in the skull are a normal variant in children, often particularly prominent between four and ten years of age, and have no clinical implications.

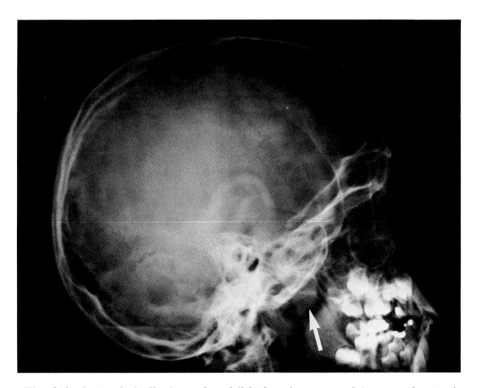

Fig. 9.4   Lateral skull view of a child showing normal 'copper-beaten' thumbprint lucencies in the frontal and occipital regions. There is also moderate prominence of the adenoidal soft tissues (arrow).

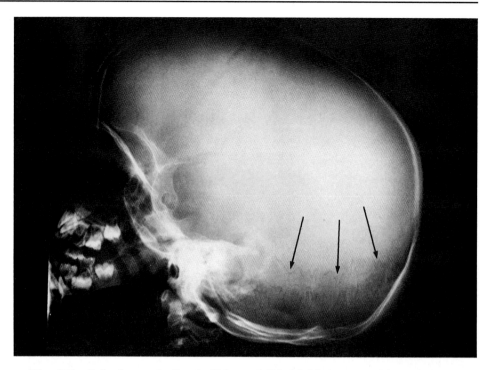

Fig. 9.5   A hydrocephalic skull in a child. Multiple wormian bones are present in the lambdoid suture (arrows).

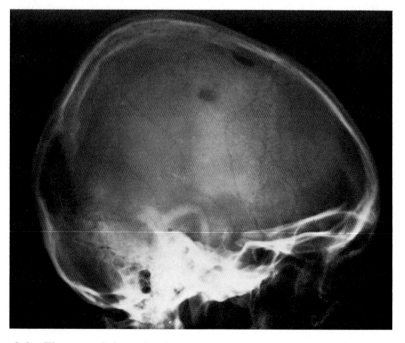

Fig. 9.6   The two defects in the parietal region are burr holes, round, well marginated and markedly transradiant due to absence of both tables.

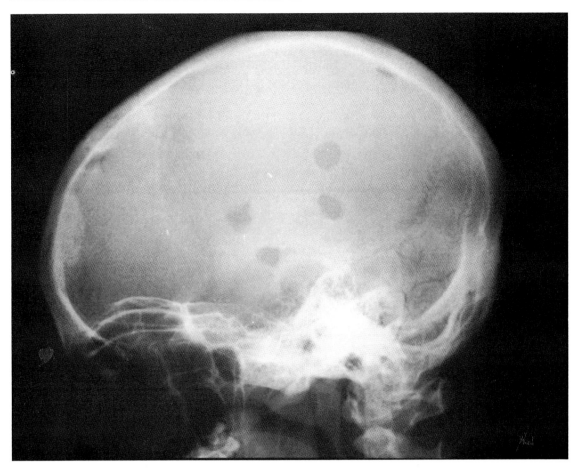

Fig. 9.7   Multiple burr holes following localization and drainage of a subdural haematoma.

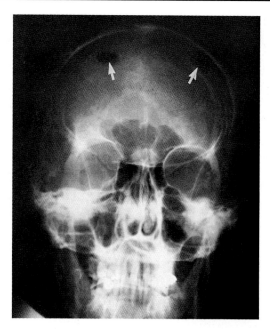

Fig. 9.8a Frontal view: bilateral burr holes (arrows) in the parietal region.

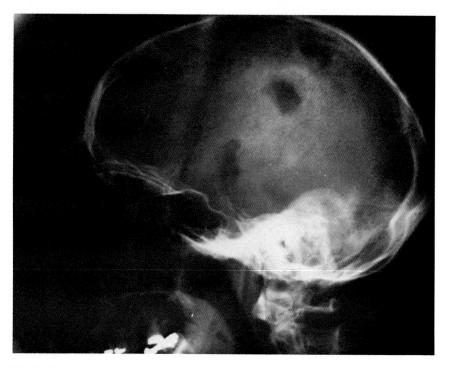

Fig. 9.8b Lateral view showing multiple burr holes and a 'nibble' taken out of the squamous temporal bone, producing very well defined skull defects.

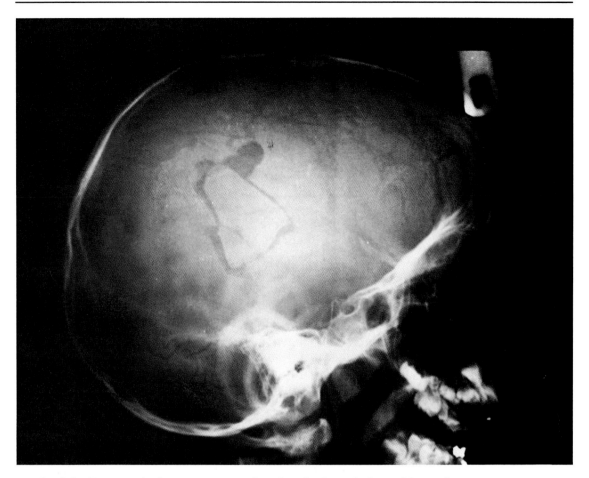

Fig. 9.9 Postsurgical appearances showing the burr hole and bone flap following drainage of a large subdural haematoma.

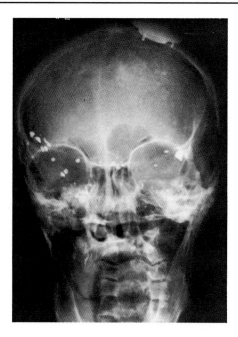

Fig. 9.10a   Frontal view showing device in left frontal region for entry in treating Parkinsonism with a stereotaxic system.

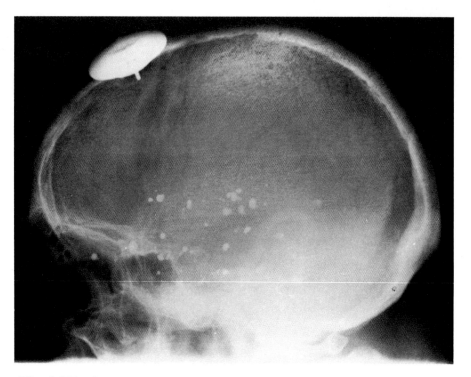

Fig. 9.10b   Lateral view showing the same surgical implant. There are also multiple opacities in the subarachnoid space due to a previous myelogram.

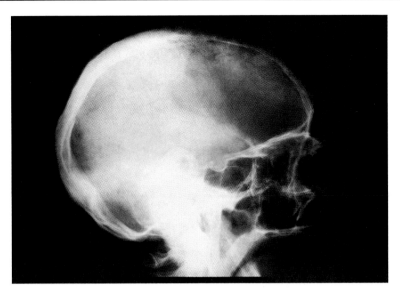

Fig. 9.11 Osteoporosis circumscripta cranialis (the early form of Paget's disease) is shown in the frontal region. The vascular grooves are still visible even though there is considerable loss of bone in the affected area. Infiltrative lesions such as metastases are not as extensive and the bone destruction obliterates the vascular pattern.

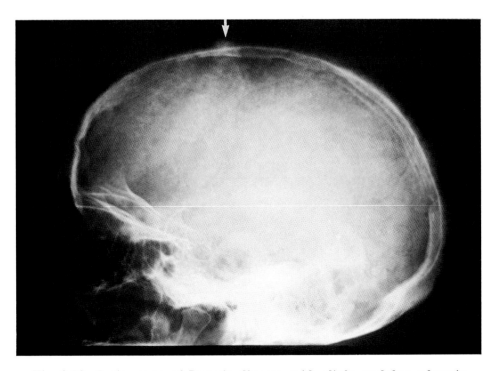

Fig. 9.12 Lytic stage of Paget's disease with slight nodular sclerotic areas; there is one prominent nodule at the apex of the frontoparietal suture (arrow) accentuated by the sclerosis around the suture.

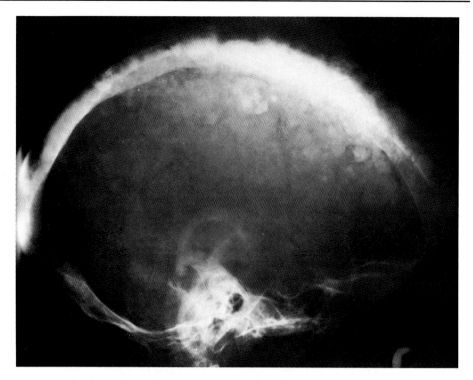

Fig. 9.13a Late Paget's disease showing the typical sclerotic nodular appearances giving a 'cotton-wool' effect. Flattening of the base of the skull, platybasia, is also present.

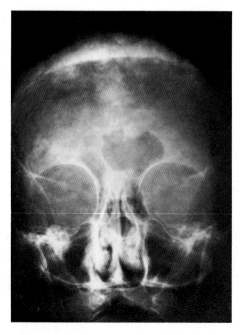

Fig. 9.13b Late Paget's disease in the frontal view in the same patient.

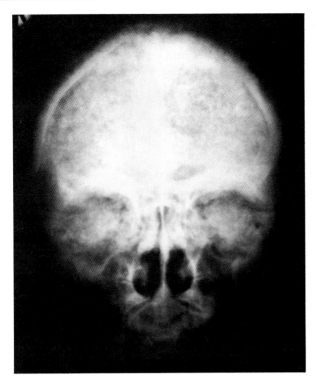

Fig. 9.14a   Gross Paget's disease showing the typical features of dense bone with multiple nodules and small lytic areas giving a 'cotton-wool' appearance.

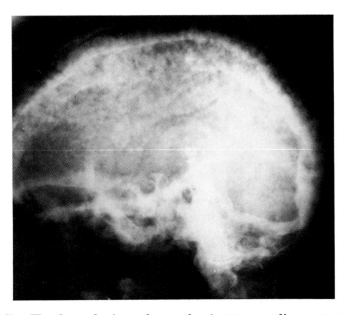

Fig. 9.14b   The lateral view shows the 'cotton-wool' appearance but there is also marked upward displacement platybasia of the skull base due to the associated bone softening.

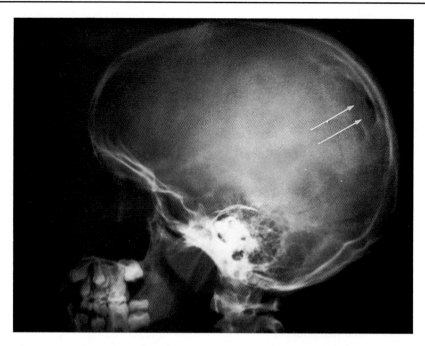

Fig. 9.15a   Large ill-defined irregular bone defect due to a metastasis (arrows).

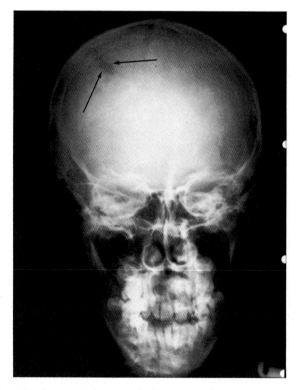

Fig. 9.15b   The lesion is less well shown on the frontal view (arrows).

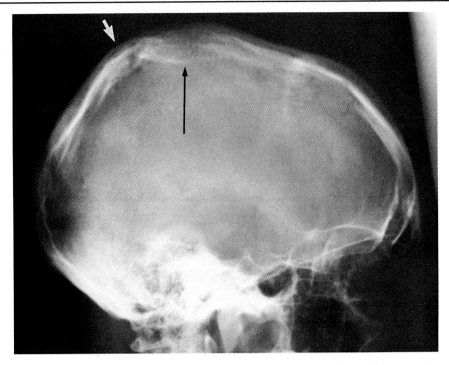

Fig. 9.16a   Thickening of the cranial vault (black arrow) and a lytic lesion lying posteriorly (white arrow).

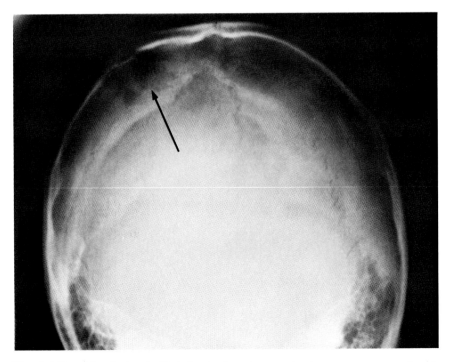

Fig. 9.16b   The lytic skull defects due to a metastases are more clearly shown on the Towne's view (arrow).

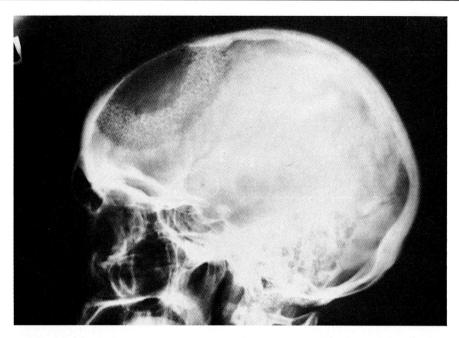

Fig. 9.17   Direct spread from a local invasive rodent ulcer. Note the pattern of erosion which has started from the outer table and do not confuse this with postoperative defect (see Fig. 9.33).

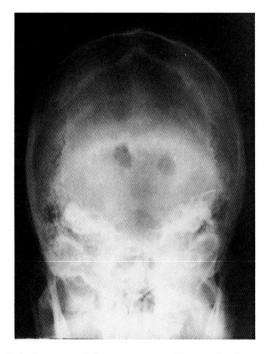

Fig. 9.18   Occipital venous lakes seen on a Towne's view, a common normal variant in the elderly. The 'lytic' lesions are bilateral, clearly defined, and close to the midline.

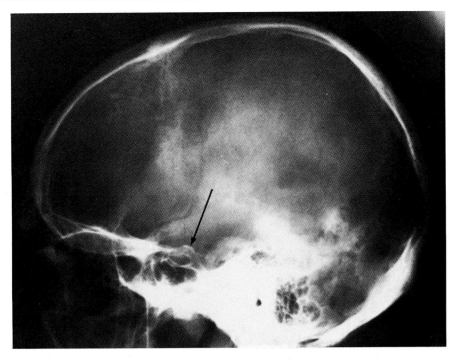

Fig. 9.19   Normal lateral view showing interclinoid calcification (arrow). A common normal variant of no clinical significance.

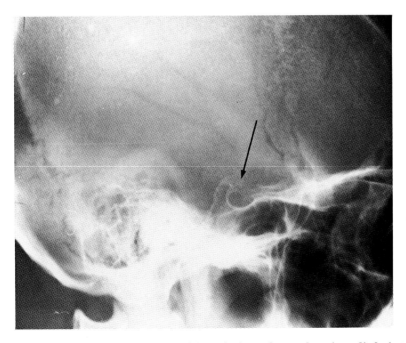

Fig. 9.20   Close-up lateral view of the pituitary fossa showing slight interclinoid calcification (arrow).

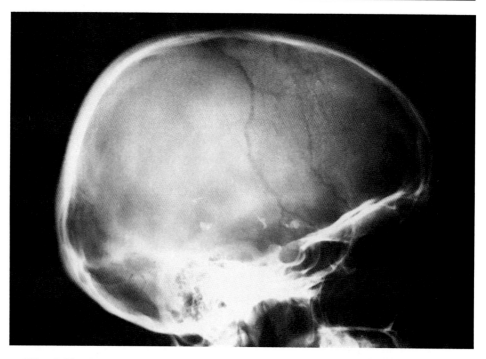

Fig. 9.21   Lateral view showing calcifications in the temporal region in a patient who had tuberculous meningitis. Do not confuse this with calcifications in the pineal gland and the choroid plexuses (see Chapter 3).

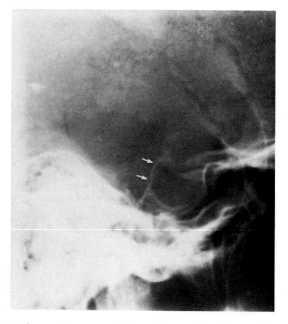

Fig. 9.22   Coned-up view on pituitary fossa showing enlarged sella with thinning of the dorsum sellae (arrows) raising the possibility of a pituitary adenoma.

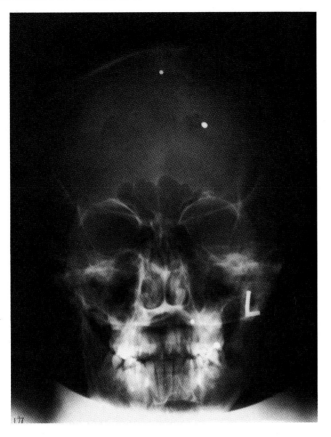

Fig. 9.23a   Flattened airgun pellets adjacent to the frontal bone in a child.

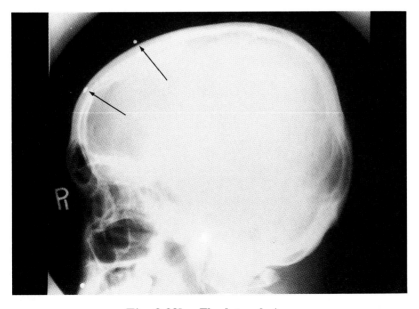

Fig. 9.23b   The lateral view.

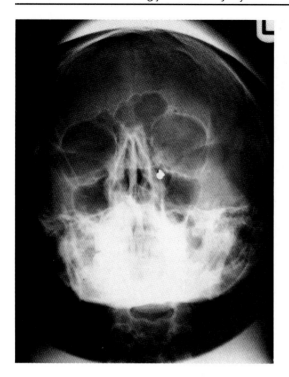

Fig. 9.24a   Airgun pellet on the left side of the face.

Fig. 9.24b   The lateral view shows the lead pellet is in the soft tissues of the upper lip.

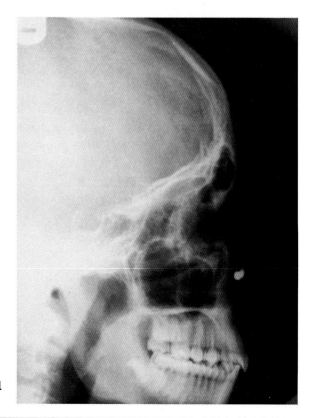

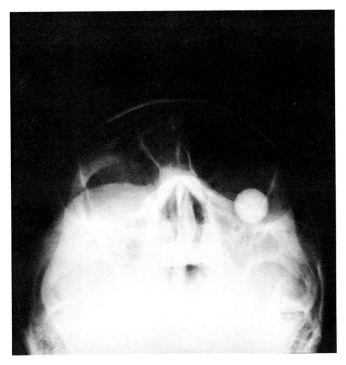

Fig. 9.25a   The round opacity on the left is a glass eye.

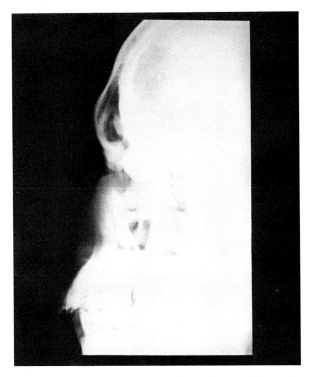

Fig. 9.25b   The lateral view localizes the opacity to the orbit.

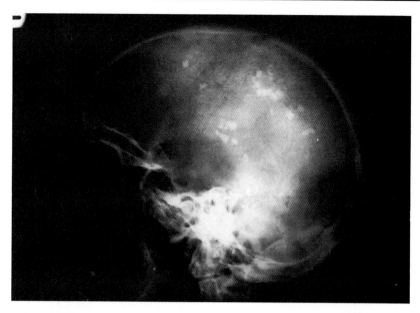

Fig. 9.26   Glass fragments trapped in the hair. Further views must be delayed until these have been removed.

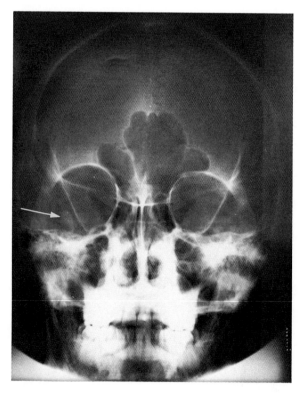

Fig. 9.27   Small glass fragment from a windscreen is lodged in the right orbit (arrow). It stresses the importance of looking carefully at the film when foreign bodies are suspected.

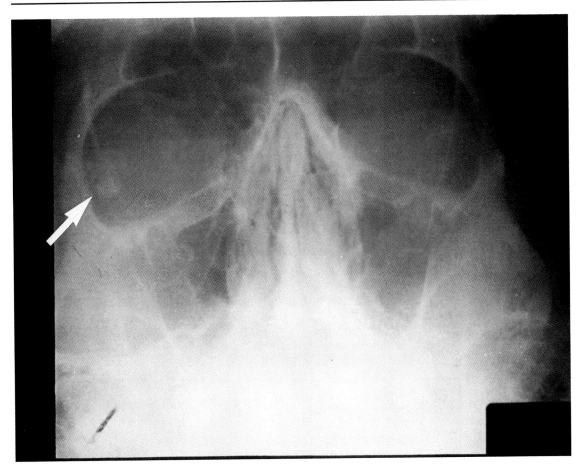

Fig. 9.28   A glass fragment (arrow) is shown in the inferolateral corner of the right orbit. Computed tomography is required for accurate localization and an assessment of the soft-tissue injury.

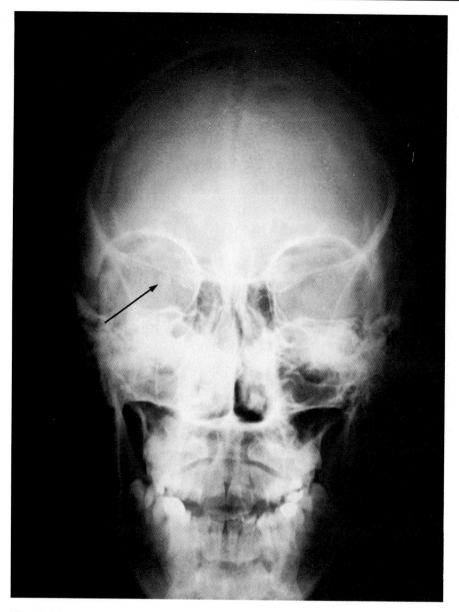

Fig. 9.29a   Glass foreign body projected over the right orbit (arrow). A further film would be required for localization.

Top right:
Fig. 9.29b   However in the Towne's view, the foreign body (arrow) is well away from the right orbit.

Below right:
Fig. 9.29c   On the lateral view, one can see the glass fragment is actually on the scalp (arrow). It is important to view the film and to locate suspected foreign bodies with a bright light.

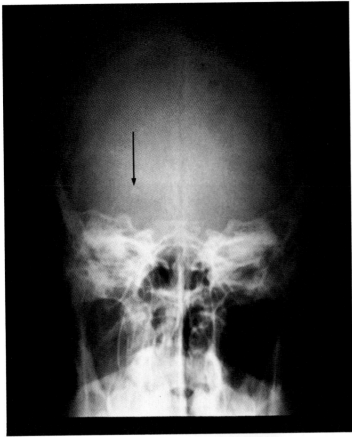

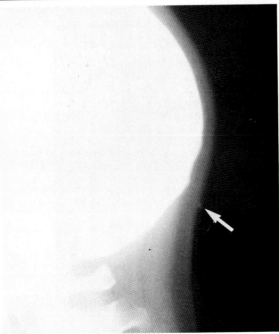

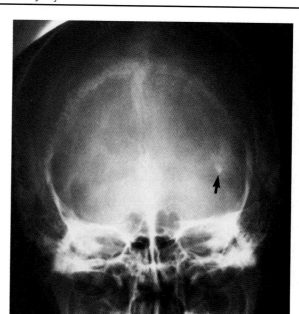

Fig. 9.30 Glass fragment (arrow) in the frontal intracranial region following a car accident.

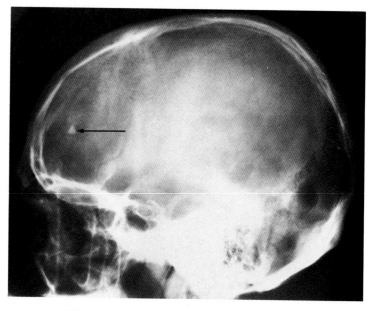

Fig. 9.31 Lateral view aids localization.

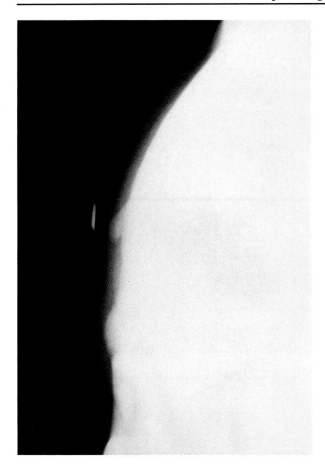

Fig. 9.32 Small glass fragment in a large frontal haematoma. The glass fragment is seen sideways on, hence it appears thin and dense.

Fig. 9.33 Postoperative defect in the frontal region with Cushing's arterial clips. A Spitz-Holter valve for ventriculovenous shunt is also present (arrow).

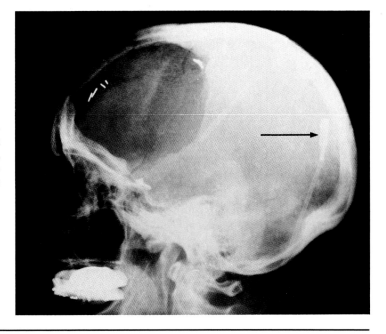

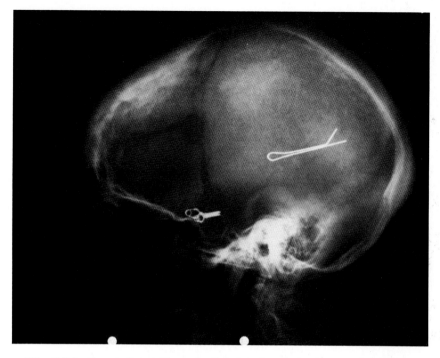

Fig. 9.34   Large frontal surgical defect but hair clips also present.

Top right:
Fig. 9.35a   Frontal view of a ventriculovenous shunt with a Spitz-Holter valve. Ventriculoperitoneal shunts are preferred in many institutions.

Below right:
Fig. 9.35b   Lateral view showing shunt in position.

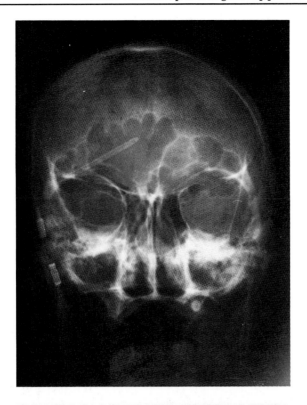

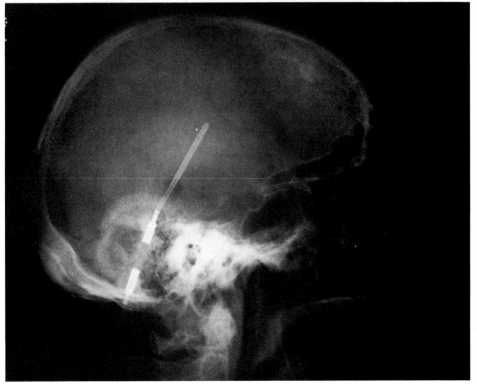

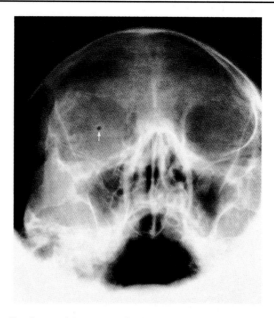

Fig. 9.36   Small ring with central air transradiancy in the right orbit (arrow) is the inner tube of a ball-point pen seen end on, lodged in the orbit.

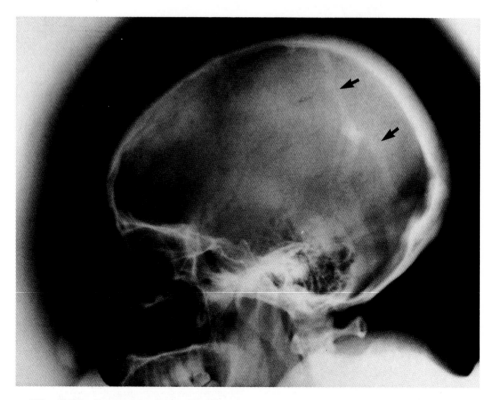

Fig. 9.37   Large markings in the posterior parietal region are thick matted hair strands clotted with blood (arrows).

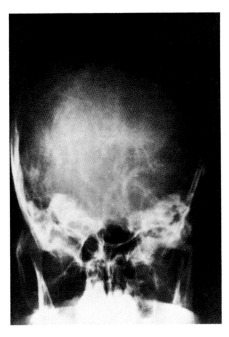

Fig. 9.38   Another example of blood in the hair showing the thick white line produced by the matted hair.

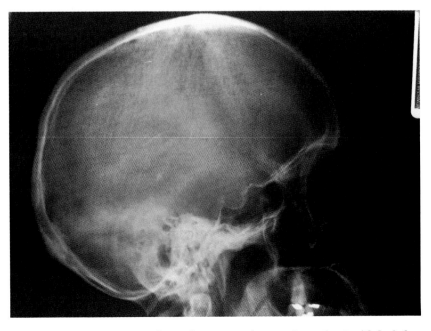

Fig. 9.39   Radiating lines from the vertex in a male patient with hair bun.

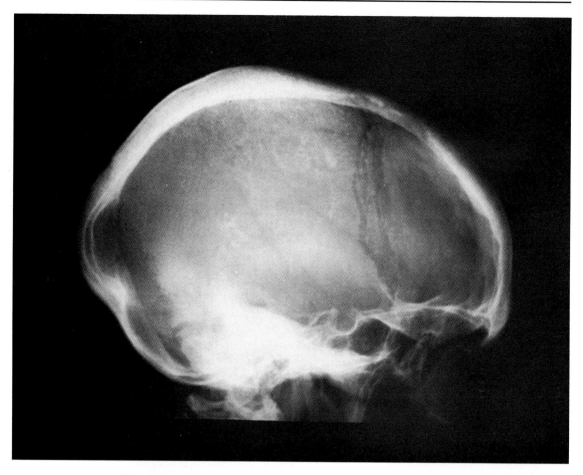

Fig. 9.40 The curvilinear lines over the superior parietal region are due to blood in the hair.

Top right:
Fig. 9.41a Towne's view of a microcephalus skull showing the small cranium secondary to craniostenosis (premature suture closure).

Below right:
Fig. 9.41b Lateral view of a microcephalic skull.

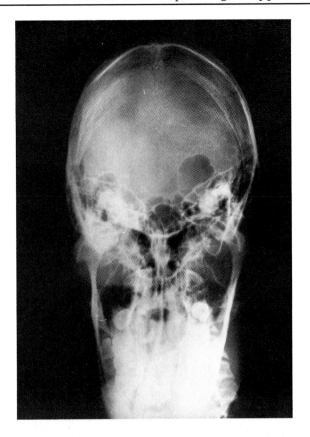

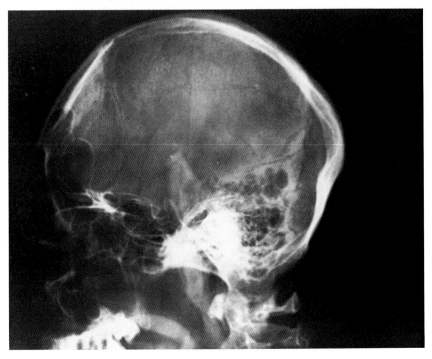

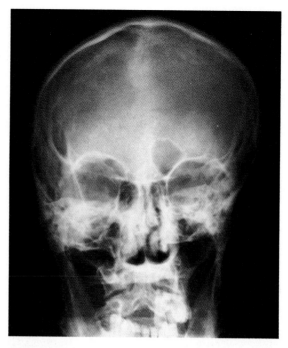

Fig. 9.42 Markedly asymmetrical cranium in an otherwise normal patient examined for skull trauma.

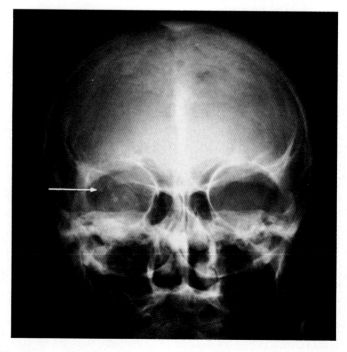

Fig. 9.43 The multiple small opacities in the right orbit (arrow) are due to phleboliths and should raise the suspicion of an angiomatous malformation.

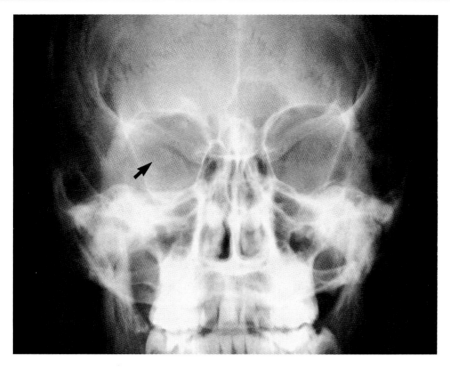

Fig. 9.44 The round opacity in the right orbit is a calcified intraocular lens (arrow) in a shrunken, atrophic blind eye.

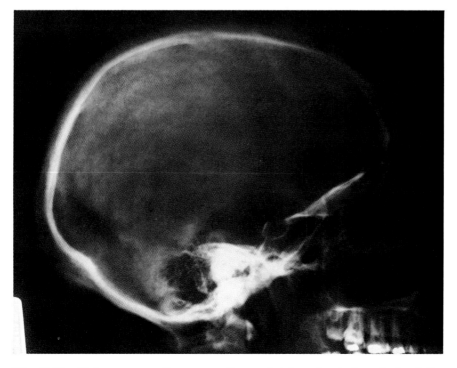

Fig. 9.45 Criss-cross pattern over the parietal region is from hair plaits.

Index